Strabismus

Strabismus

JOSEPH LANG, MD
TRANSLATED BY
GERHARD W. CIBIS, MD

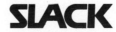

Copyright © 1984 by SLACK Incorporated

All rights reserved. No part of this book may be reproduced, stored in a retrieval system or transmitted in any form or by any means, electronic, mechanical, photocopying, recording or otherwise, without written permission from the publisher, except for brief quotations embodied in critical articles and reviews.

Printed in the United States of America

Library of Congress Catalog Card Number: 83-050673

ISBN: 0-943432-18-9

Published by: SLACK Incorporated
6900 Grove Rd.
Thorofare, NJ 08086

Last digit is print number: 8 7 6 5 4 3 2 1

Joseph Lang, MD
Professor of Ophthalmology
Director of Orthoptics and Pleoptics
University of Zurich
Switzerland

Gerhard W. Cibis, MD
Director of Clinical Ophthalmology Services
Children's Mercy Hospital
Kansas City, MO;
Associate Professor of Ophthalmology
University of Kansas
Kansas City, KS

CONTENTS

3. Types of Strabismus and Disturbances in Motility 75

TRANSLATOR'S FOREWORD

Since first published, Lang's Strabismus has fascinated me as a short, easily readable, simple yet certainly not simplistic, and, most important, nondogmatic guide to practical strabismus diagnosis and therapy. These virtues stimulated me to undertake its translation. Deviations from them are the translator's and not the author's fault. Both the experienced strabismologist and the neophyte should find this book valuable reading.

Statistics cited are based on 40,000 consecutive cases from Dr. Lang's private practice, augmented by experience derived as Director of the Ocular Motility and Orthoptic Section at the University of Zurich. Terminology used is clearly defined within the text wherever difference in usage among schools of thought might cause confusion. The reader is especially alerted to the use of microtropia, small- and large-angle esotropia, fixation point versus central scotoma and diplopia point scotoma, and the anatomy of macula, fovea, and foveola as it applies to fixation patterns.

Bangerter filters for graded occlusion therapy are available through Poll Inc., 40 W. 55th St., New York, NY, 10019, the Lang stereo test through Lang Stereo Test, P.O. Box 1413, Secaucus, NJ 07094.

I wish to thank Dr. Andrea Cibis-Tongue and Antonia Rasicovici, CO, for their review of the manuscript.

Gerhard W. Cibis, MD
Kansas City, MO

FOREWORD

D r. Lang has devoted literally his professional lifetime in ophthalmology to researching, teaching, and practicing within the subspecialty of ocular motility. His prestige in our field of work is fed from two sources. One is his thorough formal training and intimate association with respected continental colleagues, which supply that amorphous background of undisputed credibility. The other comes from within himself, identifying the emergence of a European renaissance leader in the field of strabismus for us who view the scene from another continent.

It was the author's good fortune to be born into the culture that exudes the rich heritage from which came the major portion of the classical knowledge about the anatomy, physiology, and pathology of the optical and sensorimotor systems serving vision and movement of the eyes. Dr. Lang assimilated this enormous fund of knowledge and patiently moved beyond developing new concepts that were consistent with his vast practical experience. At the same time, he was always receptive to new thoughts and techniques evolving simultaneously in other parts of the world. Old dogmas relating to strabismus procedures and teachings were questioned, and some were abandoned by him while they were still in vogue in his area and era. Yet overall he retained his continental European identity. His new thinking resulted primarily in a change of emphasis within the many nuances of our specialty—not in a radical new approach.

I have been acquainted with the author's French edition of Strabisme, Diagnostic, Formes Cliniques, Traitement, since it was published in 1981. The author's talent to convey information in an orderly manner to the student about such a complex subject struck me. The material was so logically organized, concisely explained, and well supported with clean, simple one-line drawings that it was a pleasure to read even in a language not native to me. Now, the English-speaking portion of the world is fortunate to have this book, which the author humbly refers to as a guide rather than a textbook, translated into the language with which we are most secure. Dr. Lang's methods and teachings on the subject will now be infused more readily into the everyday study and thinking of English-speaking ophthalmologists, orthoptists, and others interested in strabismus.

Regarding Dr. Lang's change in emphasis concerning the concepts and therapy of strabismus, the most notable is his keen appreciation of the fact that the majority of strabismus patients require brief inexpensive therapy, but a continuous and long follow-up. His concepts about the sensory side of strabismus led to abandonment of many of the lengthy, intense, expensive programs which by their nature discouraged long-range follow-up of the patient. His insight in this area is practical, sensitive to the patient's and family's needs, and honest in recognizing some of our limitations in influencing effectively the natural course of the disease.

Strabismus is a difficult part of ophthalmology to conquer. It affects four percent of the population. The need will always exist for good tools that impart knowledge to our colleagues who have the potential to help such a volume of afflicted people, their families, and the socioeconomic system that supports their care. Dr. Lang's input to our English-speaking professionals by way of this translated book will be a significant contribution to those who care for the large strabismus population.

Marshall M. Parks, MD
Washington, DC

1

INTRODUCTION

MOTOR

In strabismus, the visual axis of one eye is directed at the object of fixation, while the other eye deviates. In fixing a distant point, the visual axes of both eyes normally are parallel.

If one eye deviates inward, however, this is an inturning convergent strabismus, or esotropia. If it deviates out, this is divergent strabismus or exotropia. Vertical deviations are designated vertical strabismus or hypertropia (hypotropia where applicable). A vertical deviation can be isolated or can appear in combination with divergent or convergent strabismus.

When there is no manifest deviation, orthoposition or orthotropia is present. The term "parallelism" is incorrect at near gaze. One can also speak of "straight" or aligned eyes.

If the strabismus varies — sometimes the right eye deviating, other times the left eye — this is alternating strabismus. If the same eye always deviates, this is known as unilateral strabismus.

Periods of strabismus may alternate with times of normal ocular alignment. This is called intermittent strabismus, in contrast to constant strabismus.

When the angle of deviation is the same size in all directions of gaze, this is known as concomitant strabismus. In this type of strabismus, all eye muscles function normally; there is an error in the position of the eyes.

In paralytic strabismus, there is a paralysis of the nerve innervating extraocular muscle, and the angle of deviation differs with the direction of gaze according to which eye is fixing. On fixing with the sound eye, a primary angle as opposed to a secondary angle occurs with fixation with the paretic eye. The deviation is greatest in the field of action of the paralyzed muscle if the involved eye is fixing. Hence, the strabismus is incomitant. The position of the eyes is determined by anatomic and innervational factors. There are also various resting positions.

With the anatomic or absolute position of rest, there is absolutely no innervation. This occurs only in death.

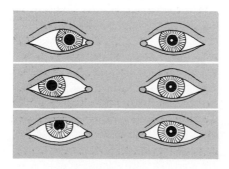

Fig. 1–
a) Convergent strabismus (esotropia) of right eye;
b) Divergent strabismus (exotropia) of left eye; and
c) Vertical strabismus (right hypertropia).

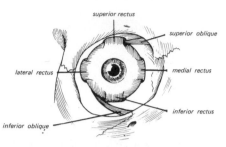

Fig. 2–Right globe; all muscles and orbit seen anteriorly.

The configuration of the orbit and its content determine the position of the eyes. The axes of the orbit are slightly deviated laterally and form an angle of about 45 degrees with each other. The resultant tendency toward divergence is increased when the orbits are even more widely separated.

The physiologic position of rest is that position in which innervation is markedly reduced and only a baseline innervational tone is present. This occurs in deep anesthesia. In this situation, it is primarily the innervation of convergence that stops, so that a divergent position is the rule. The tone of the eye muscles is highly dependent on the level of alertness and psychic orientation.

The fusion-free position of rest occurs when fusion is interrupted, as with prolonged covering of one eye. In contrast to the physiologic position of rest, all vestibular influences as well as monocular visual clues (light sensitivity, fixation) remain. Only binocularity is suspended.

An absolute parallel position, even after disruption of fusion, is called orthophoria. This is not common. After interruption of fusion, a small deviation is the rule. This is a latent strabismus or heterophoria, in contrast to a manifest strabismus or heterotropia. Esophoria, exophoria, and small degrees of hyperphoria are kept latent, and the eyes stay parallel by binocular fusion. Cyclophorias are primarily compensated for sensorially, only to a small degree by the motor system. Heterophoria can decompensate and become a manifest strabismus with loss of fusional capacity or a large latent deviation.

Primary ocular position is, with the head held straight, when the eyes are directed straight ahead onto an object at infinity. Horizontal and vertical deviations from this are known as secondary positions, oblique deviations as tertiary positions. Eye movements are carried out through the six striated external eye muscles.

The eye itself moves within Tenon's capsule almost like a ball in a ball-joint socket. The center of rotation of the globe is about 13 mm behind the cornea and 1.6 mm nasally, but it can be displaced with large eye movements. One can think of Fick's axes all going through the center of rotation. They are the transverse X, the sagittal Y, and the vertical Z axes. The equatorial plane of Listing lies on the X and Z axes. Tenon's capsule is a connective tissue shell surrounding the globe from optic nerve to limbus much like a joint capsule.

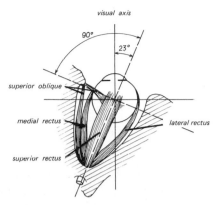

Fig. 3–Right eye, muscles, and orbit as viewed from above.

Eye movements of up to 45 degrees are possible to either side and down, but are possible only to 30 degrees on upgaze. Greater movements are hindered by the optic nerves and check ligaments. Check ligaments are particularly prominent on the internal and external recti, and they connect Tenon's capsule with the bony orbital wall.

The four straight eye muscles, namely the medial rectus, superior rectus, inferior rectus, and lateral rectus, are all 40 to 41 mm in length. They originate at the tendinous annulus of Zinn at the optic canal. Their tendinous insertions are 4 to 8 mm long and about 1 mm wide and insert into the sclera 5.5 to 7 mm from the limbus. The distance between the muscle insertion and the limbus increases from the medial rectus (5.5 mm) to the inferior rectus (6.5 mm) and from the lateral rectus (6.9 mm) to the superior rectus (7.7 mm). This forms the spiral of Tillaux. The shortest tendon is that of the medial rectus, being 3.8 mm, and the longest is that of the lateral rectus, at 8.8 mm.

The medial rectus is an adductor. Its antagonist, the lateral rectus, is an abductor. Both are pure horizontal motor muscles. The superior and inferior recti are primarily vertical motor muscles. Since their course runs 23 degrees divergent from straight ahead, they only work as pure vertical motor muscles when the globe is abducted to this degree. When the globe is adducted, the superior rectus functions as an intorter, the inferior rectus as an extorter. The oblique depressor, the superior oblique muscle, also has its origin at the tendinous annulus of Zinn and courses 40 mm to the trochlea, which is positioned slightly above the inner angle of the lid and is attached to the bony orbital rim. In the 10 mm leading to the trochlea, the muscle constricts into a tendon, which courses through the trochlea then angulates sharply to run posteriorly beneath the superior rectus muscle to insert broadly in the upper temporal quadrant of the globe behind the equator. The superior oblique muscle is 60 mm in length, of which 30 mm is muscle and 30 mm tendon.

The superior rectus muscle forms an angle of 23 degrees with the visual axis. Its maximum elevating action occurs when the globe is abducted 23 degrees. The superior oblique muscle forms an angle of 55 degrees with the visual axis. Its maximal action as a depressor occurs when the eye is adducted to this degree. At 35 degrees of abduction, the superior oblique is a pure intorter.

The oblique elevator, the inferior oblique, is the only muscle that does not originate at the orbital apex. It arises at the nasal rim of the bony orbital floor. From there it courses beneath the inferior rectus and angles laterally and posteriorly to insert onto the globe near the macula and the posterior inferior quadrant. It is 35 mm in length. The region where it crosses the inferior rectus is known as Lockwood's ligament. The globe rests on Lockwood's ligament like it is in a hammock.

TABLE 1–1.

LENGTH OF EXTRAOCULAR MUSCLES AND TENDONS

	Muscle	Tendon	Total
M. rectus sup.	41.8 mm	5.8 mm	46.8 mm
M. rectus inf.	40 mm	5.5 mm	46.5 mm
M. rectus medialis	40.8 mm	3.8 mm	44.8 mm
M. rectus lateralis	40.6 mm	8.8 mm	49.8 mm
M. obliquus sup.	30 mm	10+20 mm	60.0 mm
M. obliquus inf.	37 mm	1 mm	38 mm

In abduction, the superior oblique acts primarily as an intorter; in adduction, as a depressor. Its antagonist, the inferior oblique, functions as an extorter in abduction and as an elevator in adduction. The abducting function of the oblique is of minimal significance.

The tendon of the superior oblique forms an angle of 55 degrees with the visual axis. The inferior oblique tendon forms an angle of 51 degrees with the visual axis. The course of the superior oblique therefore is somewhat more transverse than that of the inferior oblique, which is more sagittal. This small difference in the axis of the oblique muscles results in the antagonistic action of the two obliques, which are not always totally balanced. The elevating action of the inferior oblique is stronger than the depressing action of the superior oblique, particularly in adduction.[80] It must be remembered that all these numbers are averages, and as shown by Fink, great variations are possible especially among the oblique muscles. Monocular eye movements are called ductions. Adduction or inturning results from action of the internal rectus, whereas abduction is carried out by its antagonist, the external rectus.

In elevation, also called sursumduction, the superior rectus and inferior oblique behave synergistically. Depression, or deorsumduction, is carried out by the inferior rectus and the superior oblique.

Extorsion, also called excycloduction, is primarily the function of the inferior oblique, with some assistance from the inferior rectus. In intorsion, or incycloduction, the superior oblique is assisted by the superior rectus.

The eye muscles, like skeletal muscles, follow Sherrington's law of reciprocal innervation. With contraction of an agonist, the antagonist relaxes. For example, when the superior rectus muscle contracts, the inferior rectus relaxes. This relationship can be demonstrated with electromyography.

Humans are unable to move one eye independent of the other. This is unlike some animals such as the chameleon, which is able to move each eye separately. Binocular ocular movements are differentiated into those having a similarity of direction — called conjugate eye movements or ductions — and those with opposite direction, called disconjugate eye movement or vergences.

Hering's law applies to the eyes as a team. It states that in conjugate movements, innervation goes equally to synergistic muscles in each eye. For example, on right gaze the lateral rectus of the right eye receives the same strength of innervational impulses as the medial rectus of the left eye. In this way, perfectly balanced movements of both eyes occur. This law is of particular importance in paralysis of eye muscles. With conjugate eye movements, there are always two muscles that act synergistically; for

Fig. 4-Schema of the action of the extraocular muscles in primary position (after Marquez).

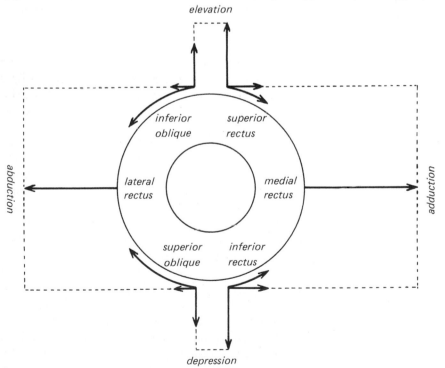

example, on right gaze these are the right lateral rectus and the left medial rectus.

The primary action of the oblique muscles is torsion; that of the vertical recti is vertical movement. The horizontal action of these muscles is minimal. The internal rectus and the lateral rectus have purely horizontal functions. Disconjugate eye movements are called vergences, the most important of which is convergence. Its opposite is divergence. Contrary to convergence, voluntary divergence does not seem to exist. Instead, a relaxation of convergence is a more-or-less passive event. Fusional divergence, however, does exist, and vertical vergences are possible. With vertical convergence movements, the eyes move closer to each other in their vertical position, whereas with vertical divergence movement, the vertical separation increases. With cyclovergence movements, one must differentiate between incyclovergence and excyclovergence. Fusional torsion movement balances out cyclophoria.

To understand the function of eye muscles, one must know their microscopic ultrastructure.[97] Whereas 140 muscle fibers are innervated by one nerve fiber in skeletal muscles, in the eye muscles one nerve fiber innervates 10 muscle fibers. There are two types of muscle fibers: (1) The central muscle fibers in the belly of the muscle have a large diameter, with a fibrillar structure, and react with rapid contraction movements following the all-or-nothing law. They are innervated by rapid-conducting myelin-sheathed alpha nerve fibers. (2) Muscle fibers in the muscle periphery have a field structure and primarily react to excitation with a slow tonic contracture. They are innervated by more delicate and slower conducting nonmyelin-sheathed gamma nerve fibers.

Only the discharge of alpha motor neurons is recorded with electromyography. Discharge of the gamma motor neurons, which are of particular importance in concomitant strabismus, is not registered.[51] The oculomotor nerve innervates the superior, medial, and inferior recti as well as the inferior oblique muscles. The levator palpebral muscle of the lid is also innervated by the oculomotor nerve. Accommodation is made possible by parasympathetic fibers of the oculomotor nerve, which reach the ciliary muscle via the ciliary ganglion.

The trochlear nerve innervates only a single eye muscle, the superior oblique. The abducens nerve innervates only the lateral rectus.

The nuclear region of the oculomotor nerve is in the brain stem at the level of the aqueduct of Sylvius. Caudal to this lies the nucleus of the trochlear nerve. The abducens nucleus lies further back, in the floor of the fourth ventricle.

Disturbances in the nuclear or infranuclear region lead to paralysis of single or multiple eye muscles. Supranuclear disturbances cause difficulty in coordination and, as a rule, affect both eyes equally, causing gaze paresis. The various nuclei are joined and coordinated through the posterior longitudinal fasciculus. The posterior and longitudinal fasciculi also serve to conduct impulses from the vestibular nerve and from subcortical centers to produce horizontal eye movements.

Impulses for voluntary eye movement originate in the frontal cortex, where there is a center for voluntary eye movements. A second cortical center for eye movements is in the occipital lobe adjacent to the visual cortex. All optically evoked impulses for eye movement originate here. This includes the fixation mechanisms, the fusional mechanisms, and the accommodative processes as well as visual following movements.

The vestibular apparatus has a stabilizing influence on ocular motility. Every change in position of the head or body leads to compensatory eye movements via statokinetic reflexes.

The nature of eye movements varies with and is characteristic of the mechanism evoking them. Fixation movements or saccades are very quick. Horizontal saccades originate in the parapontine reticular formation (PPRF) adjacent to the abducens nucleus. Vertical saccades originate in the mesencephalic reticular formation adjacent to the ocular motor nerve nuclei. Visual following movements are markedly slower. The slowest is the system for fusional movements.

Fig. 5–Schema for the higher centers of eye movement. Voluntary eye movements originate in the frontal gaze center (A). From the occipital gaze center come impulses for eye movement evoked by visual stimuli (B). The vestibular system sends impulses through the nucleus of the eighth nerve (C). It is connected by the posterior longitudinal fasciculus to the nuclei of the extraocular muscles.

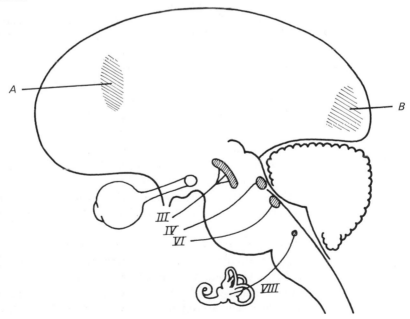

A simple experiment shows how much more rapid the vestibular ocular motor system works than, for example, the mechanism for visual following movements. Rapidly move a page of print up and down and attempt to read. The text is blurred. Now hold the text still and at the same speed as previously make vertical head movements. Reading is now possible.

The exact connecting pathways for supranuclear centers are only partially known. Relatively little is also known about the spontaneous activity from the brain stem, psychologic influences on ocular motility (increase in angle of deviation with embarrassment, anger, or fear), and proprioception from the eye muscle. It is therefore not surprising that there is not a satisfactory explanation for many eye muscle movement disorders.

Even today, one still speaks of reflexes. For example, "fixation reflex" or "fusion reflex" and "reflex for binocular vision" are used in referring to the sensory and motor aspects of vision. The term "reflex" may be adequate for simple events such as the patellar reflex. In the visual process, however, one is dealing with a much more complicated interaction of various mechanisms evoked by external stimuli and influenced by the internal activity of the central nervous system. Visual "reflexes" may be learned or with practice may become interconnected. An understanding of these complex events is easier if one does not think strictly in reflex terminology but more in the sense of a steering or regulatory system such as a feedback mechanism.

SENSORY

NORMAL BINOCULAR VISION

Normal binocular vision should be discussed in order to understand the various sensory changes that occur with strabismus. This is best done with an example.

Figure 6 shows as fixation objects a church and an adjacent tree. Attention is directed to the church tower. What time is it?

On the fundus, this picture is reversed both vertically and horizontally (Fig. 7). The object of fixation — the church tower clock — is projected onto the fovea, the point of sharpest vision. The other objects appear on the retina to either side of the macula at various intervals. Every retinal point, meaning the smallest retinal area, has a directional value. The fovea has the direction of straight ahead. It therefore represents the primary visual direction. With it we look directly at an object. The remaining retinal points form the surrounding area. A point beneath the fovea has the directional value of just above straight ahead. A point nasal to the fovea has the directional value of temporal from straight ahead. The relationship of objects to each other in space, for example, tree to church tower, is called relative localization. The relationship of objects to the observer is called "absolute" or "egocentric localization." Cooperation between the two eyes is based on the fact that the visual fields of each eye overlap and that in each eye, points or areas with the same directional value are found. These points are called "corresponding retinal points." In the past, one spoke of retinal identity or congruence; one now speaks of correspondence.

Retinal correspondence can be demonstrated by the experiment of Hering. Stand about 50 cm in front of a window so that you can see two distinct objects, for example, a tree and a chimney. On the window pane, mark a dot that without moving the head will cover the tree when the right eye is fixing and the chimney when the left eye is fixing. If you look at the dot with both eyes, the tree and chimney are perceived to be in the same direction, although they are not. The foveas of both eyes have the same directional value.

An even simpler way of demonstrating retinal correspondence is to fixate a light with one eye and to project the star figure of an ophthalmoscope into the other. When the light and star are superimposed, both objects are imaged on the fovea. One can then displace the star a specific distance from the fixation

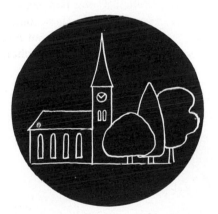

Fig. 6–Fixation picture.

Fig. 7–Projection onto the fundus with eyes parallel.

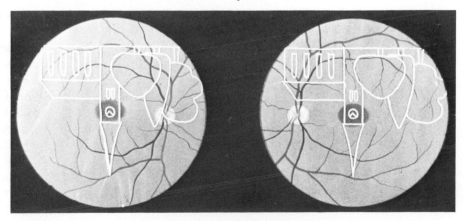

light and thereby determine the correspondence value of adjacent retinal areas, as on a coordinate system.

With binocular vision, both eyes have corresponding points with the same visual direction. Retinal points stimulated by the same impulses are called "corresponding retinal points." The pictures from both retinas are integrated in the visual cortex into a single visual impression. This is called cyclopic sensation or a cyclopian eye, which is subjectively localized to the base of the nose.

The horopter represents the points in space corresponding to the retina. This is an imaginary surface in space whose center is the object of fixation. Only points that lie on the surface of the horopter stimulate corresponding retinal points. Points in front of or behind the surface of the horopter are referred to as physiologic diplopia. The theoretic or geometric horopter lies on a circle that runs through the point of fixation and the nodal points to the pupils of both eyes. This is differentiated from the experimental or empiric horopter, which is flatter than the theoretic. Its form changes with the distance of observation. At a distance of two meters, it forms a frontal parallel straight line. Further than two meters, its form is convex; closer than two meters, it is concave.

Fig. 8–Horopter (*H*); Panum's area (*P*).

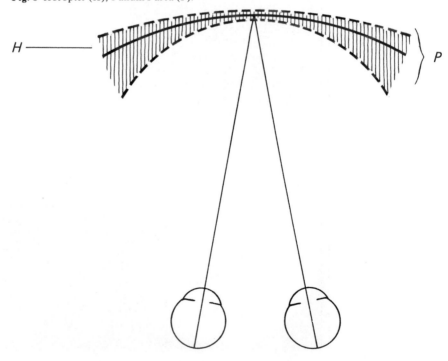

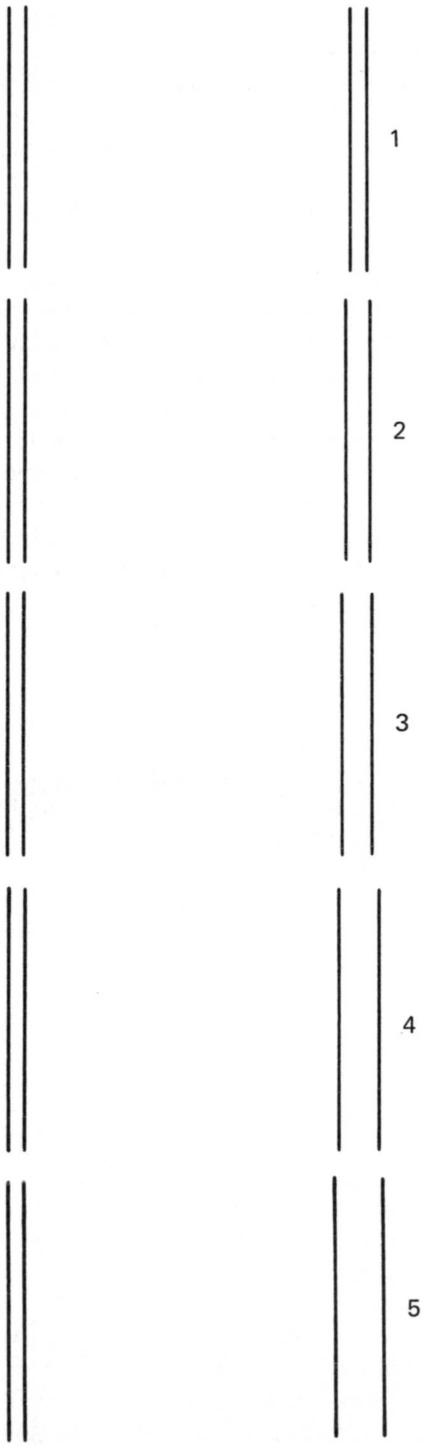

Fig. 9A–Panum's experiment to demonstrate stereoscopic vision through angular disparity.
1. Both lines equal in size, as are all the lines in the left-hand column.
2. Lines on the right are 1 mm further apart.
3. Lines on the right are 2 mm further apart.
4. Lines on the right are 3 mm further apart.
5. Lines on the right are 4 mm further apart.

Stereopsis is possible with 2., 3., and 4. With 5., it is no longer possible, and three lines are seen.

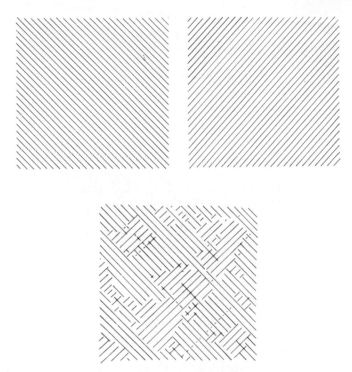

Fig. 9B–Panum's demonstration of suppression (retinal rivalry). The diagonal lines are not fused but suppressed in a mosaiclike fashion.

Investigations on the stereoscope show that pictures that are not totally identical can still be integrated into a single visual image. This results in a sense of stereopsis. This led Panum to reexamine the concept of corresponding retinal points.[110] He found that corresponding retinal areas are not pointlike in nature but have a certain range. He presented two vertical lines to each eye and changed the distance of these lines to the eye in a stepwise fashion. When both pairs of lines are at the same distance from the eyes, there is no sense of depth. If the distance of one of the pairs is changed slightly, a sensation of depth develops. If it is changed markedly, the lines may be seen double. This is known as Panum's area. In the retinal center, it is approximately five minutes of arc and enlarges into the periphery. Panum's area of the retina corresponds in space to an expansion of the horopter anteriorly and posteriorly.

Diplopia results if similar visual objects lie outside Panum's area. To alleviate this, a motor movement must occur to correct the eye position. The eye muscles are able to direct both eyes exactly onto the object of fixation. Fusion, therefore, has a sensory and a motor component.

SUPPRESSION

Rivalry between the two visual perceptions occurs when each eye is presented with a dissimilar picture. This is best illustrated with an example designed by Panum. If the right eye looks at a square with diagonal lines running in one direction, and the left eye looks at a square with diagonal lines running at a right angle to those presented to the right eye, then no fusion of the two images develops, only retinal rivalry. Over time, that picture to which attention is directed dominates, while the other picture is suppressed. A normal example of this familiar to all of us occurs with monocular microscopy. This suppression primarily involves the retinal center. The strabismic child reacts the same way but to a much greater extent.

In the strabismic patient, a shift of the image occurs on the fundus. Figure 10 shows this condition in an esotropia of 17 degrees. In the right eye, which fixes straight ahead, the visual image falls directly on the fovea. In the left eye, it is shifted 17 degrees nasally, onto a retinal point next to the optic disc. The fovea of the strabismic eye is stimulated by a different image, in this example, a tree. Whereas the right eye has the impression that the church tower clock is straight ahead, the strabismic eye perceives the tree as being straight ahead. This results in confusion — the superimposition of two objects in the same place. Since the strabismic eye sees the church tower as being left of straight ahead, diplopia develops — the same object is in two places. To avoid this disturbance, the strabismic eye is suppressed.

Adults with paralytic strabismus complain of diplopia, which is very disturbing. In children, diplopia is rarely expressed. Only when strabismus develops suddenly after three years of age will some children spontaneously express diplopia, which disappears quickly.

The suppression zones vary in different parts of the retina. The macula is strongly suppressed because it is the area of sharpest vision; therefore, the occurrence of a double image in this region would be the most disturbing. This area of suppression in the macular region would be more appropriately called macular or foveal scotoma. It can be of varying intensity and diameters. The second suppression zone exists in the area where the image stimulating the macula of the fixing eye stimulates that of the deviating eye. This is called diplopia point scotoma or null point scotoma or, as according to Harms, a fixation point scotoma.[60] One must differentiate precisely whether a scotoma occurs only with monocular vision or is limited to the binocular visual field. The term "central scotoma with monocular viewing" denotes a foveal or macular scotoma. With binocular vision, the term "central scotoma" denotes not a foveal but a null point scotoma (or diplopia or fixation point scotoma).

Investigation of two different types of strabismus, namely monocular and alternating, for evidence of suppression reveals the following: With alternating strabismus, the areas of suppression alternate from one eye to the other.

With the left eye fixing, the right eye is suppressed. After shifting fixation to the right eye, the visual impulse to the left eye is suppressed. Suppression is a labile mechanism. With monocular strabismus, the same eye is always suppressed, and its visual function is therefore markedly depressed. The foveal scotoma and the null point scotoma increase in size and intensity. What at first was a labile condition turns into a stable one. The suppression mechanism is no longer reversible. There is a decline in visual function in this eye, which leads to strabismic amblyopia.

ANOMALOUS RETINAL CORRESPONDENCE (ARC)

There is a second adaptation to strabismus for binocular vision in addition to suppression. This is anomalous retinal correspondence. Anomalous retinal correspondence occurs when noncorresponding retinal points have the same sense of visual direction.

It is well known that every retinal point has its specific sense of direction. If in the left eye, a point nasal to the fovea is stimulated, this is interpreted as left of straight ahead. If the point stimulated is beneath the fovea, it is seen as above straight ahead. In binocular vision, only corresponding retinal points have the same sense of direction. This is illustrated in Figure 7.

In strabismus with anomalous retinal correspondence during binocular vision, the sensory direction of the deviating eye is displaced appropriately in the direction of the angle of deviation. The subjective sensation of straight ahead for the deviating eye is no longer at the fovea but in the region nasal to the disc (Fig. 10).

Theoretically, this area of the deviating eye has the same visual direction as the fovea of the fixing eye. It is therefore called the localization center of anomalous correspondence — pseudo macula.[136] The simplest term is "anomaly center." Other retinal areas are oriented around this center.

In the cerebral cortex, instead of the usually corresponding retinal points, the anomalous corresponding retinal points are now unified into a single image. In this way, the strabismic patient achieves binocularity without diplopia. This aberration of the directional sense of the strabismic eye exists only as long as both eyes are open. With monocular or alternating vision, the sense of direction for "straight ahead" returns to the foveola in cases of central fixation. In case of eccentric fixation, the binocular and monocular visual direction sense may be the same, but usually the point of eccentric fixation is closer to the foveola than the center of anomalous retinal correspondence.

In practice, not only is there usually a shift in the sense of direction in the deviating eye (anomalous retinal correspondence), but also this anomalous retinal correspondence is usually combined with suppression of varying degrees. The suppression zone in the deviating eye primarily lies in that area of the retina anomalously corresponding to the macula of the leading eye.

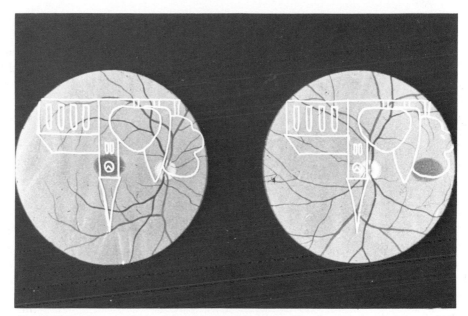

Fig. 10–Projection onto the fundi in esotropia of 17 degrees. The church tower clock is nasal to the disc.

This suppression scotoma therefore usually affects the localization center of anomalous retinal correspondence and is called the null point scotoma or fixation point scotoma of Harms. The term "diplopia point scotoma" is not precisely correct here, because with anomalous retinal correspondence there is no diplopia in this area.

With the synoptophore, with its arms at the subjective angle, this fixation point scotoma appears as suppression or jumping of pictures. With Bagolini lenses, it is a gap seen by the deviating eye in the streak of light near the fixation light. One can do direct perimetry of this zero point or fixation point scotoma in the fundus by testing bifoveally. One must keep fixation point scotoma in mind during examination in order to define anomalous retinal correspondence. The following definition, which appears primarily in the English-speaking literature, is too restricted: "Anomalous correspondence is a binocular condition whereby the macula of the fixing eye is used with a retinal point other than the macula in the nonfixing eye."

By this definition, an anomalous retinal correspondence is less common than by our definition, since the point corresponding to the macula is usually suppressed. One must view anomalous retinal correspondence as a relationship between visual fields rather than between points. The center of anomaly even when suppressed represents the center of anomalous retinal correspondence on a coordinated system.

Examination within this area of scotoma also leads to the erroneous belief that fusion and stereopsis are not possible with anomalous retinal correspon-

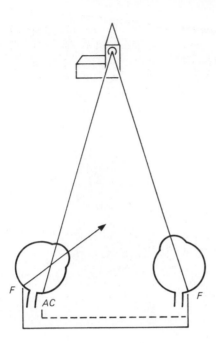

Fig. 11–Left esotropia. With normal retinal correspondence, both foveae correspond (F-F).

With anomalous retinal correspondence, the fovea of the right eye and the anomaly center of the left eye (AC) have the same sense of visual direction.

dence. If one uses sufficiently large test objects that extend outside the suppression scotoma, fusional movements and depth perception can be elicited.

As a rule, retinal correspondence is harmonious. This means that despite a manifest angle of deviation, subjectively the angle is zero. The angle of anomaly corresponds to the angle of deviation.

With unharmonious abnormal retinal correspondence, the subjective angle is not zero degrees. When unharmonious anomalous retinal correspondence is found, this can usually be explained as a testing artifact. At the synoptophore, for example, it is common for a convergent angle of 12 degrees to increase to 18 degrees. Subjectively, the images are then seen not at zero degrees but at +6 degrees owing to instrument convergence. Similarly, the angle of convergence increases with the dark red glass. This is then also misinterpreted as an unharmonious anomalous retinal correspondence. A true unharmonious anomalous retinal correspondence, however, is expected immediately following a change in the angle of deviation; for example, after strabismus surgery. This can lead to paradoxic diplopia. For example, an angle of 15 degrees is reduced to zero — objectively straight, but subjectively interpreted as a divergence of 15 degrees.

Anomalous retinal correspondence is not very stable and often is variable, corresponding to the angle of deviation. For example, in a "V" pattern the angle of anomaly may be larger looking down than looking up, while the sensory adaptation harmoniously adjusts itself to the angle of deviation.[26]

It is said that anomalous correspondence may alternate with normal correspondence in the same patient. An example is intermittent exotropia, in which the eyes are parallel with normal correspondence at near gaze, but anomalous retinal correspondence occurs with divergence on far gaze. We, however, have not seen this relationship even once.

In a sense, one can consider anomalous correspondence as "internal strabismus." The external strabismus is recognized by the deviant positions of the two eyes, and internal strabismus by the sensory retinal adaptation to this position. The oculomotor movements are then secondarily coupled to this anomalous retinal correspondence.

It is generally assumed that anomalous retinal correspondence is a sensory adaptation to the strabismic position. It is a condition that is acquired in the first few years of life. Anomalous retinal correspondence is rare in strabismus developing after three years of age.

In our cases of microtropia, we have seen that there is probably a hereditary predilection for anomalous retinal correspondence. This is usually in the form of a primary ultrasmall-angle strabismus. If the angle of deviation then increases for any reason, the anomalous retinal correspondence will adapt itself to this new eye position.

Since 85% of all children with concomitant esotropia show anomalous retinal correspondence, this is of great practical significance for diagnosis and treatment.

AMBLYOPIA

The word "amblyopia" comes from the Greek word for "equal and dull" and signifies weak vision.

The word "amblyopia" occurred in the writings of Hippocrates, where it signified weak vision without further explanation. Plenk in 1788 defined amblyopia as weak vision without visible ocular damage as the cause. For Plenk, strabismus was the result of amblyopia, not its cause.[118]

Without using the term "amblyopia," Buffon in 1743 advocated occlusion as treatment for decreased vision associated with strabismus. He believed that with improvement in vision, the strabismus would also be cured.[17]

At present, the word "amblyopia" is only rarely used in connection with organically caused decreases in vision, such as tobacco-alcohol amblyopia or quinine amblyopia. Usually, amblyopia is considered to be functional, meaning reversible, and one therefore speaks quite correctly of a functional amblyopia. If there is a combination of organic and functional causes, one speaks of "a mixed amblyopia." It is not always possible to decide whether amblyopia is purely functional. However, when vision loss is reversible by exercises, this is proof of the functional nature of this amblyopia.

There are various types of amblyopia (amblyopia ex anisometropia, strabismic amblyopia, amblyopia ex anopsia, and so forth) and many factors leading to amblyopia (lack of fixation, suppression mechanism, or blurred image), which may appear singly or in combination. Neurophysiologically,

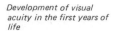

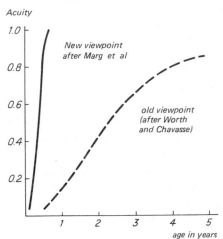

Development of visual
acuity in the first years of
life

Acuity

New viewpoint
after Marg et al

old viewpoint
(after Worth
and Chavasse)

age in years

Fig. 12–Development of visual acuity during the first years of life.
a) New concepts according to Marg et al;
b) Old concept after Worth and Chavasse.

amblyopia is by no means understood. It therefore seems useful to describe the clinical appearance of various types in a stepwise fashion.

It must be understood from the outset that vision develops in the first years of life. The macula is anatomically not differentiated until four months of age. The acellular layer of Chievitz is still found there at this time. It was formerly thought that full visual acuity was not reached until three to five years of age. New investigations have shown, however, that a visual acuity of 1.0 is possible by the age of six to eight months. Binocular vision also develops more rapidly than previously thought. Visual evoked potentials have demonstrated stereopsis as early as six months of age. Only subsequently is there a slow improvement in visual resolution. Intelligent children without refractive errors can see 20/20 by three years of age.

BILATERAL AMETROPIC AMBLYOPIA

Decreased visual acuity is common with high bilateral refractive errors; for example, uncorrected astigmatism. It is typical of astigmatism that the uncorrected visual acuity is fairly good but fails to improve significantly with glasses when first prescribed. Generally, uncorrected acuity can be 0.3 (20/70) in spite of an astigmatism of 3 diopters. Less astigmatism gives better vision; more severe astigmatism is associated with a vision of 0.1 (20/200) or 0.2 (20/100). A refractive correction improves vision only minimally at first. Full correction is often rejected, and the optimal subjective correction is difficult to determine. In the beginning, these children do not appreciate any benefit from glasses and therefore do not wear them. Only after a month or two, sometimes after as many as two years, of wearing glasses is the final visual acuity reached.

It appears that the blurred visual impressions are utilized in an optimal way by the patient. The astigmatic correction requires a major reorientation of the patient's visual behavior.

One can interpret the decreased vision with astigmatism as a form of retarded development. Full visual acuity could not develop, since the retina never was presented with a clear image. With the glasses, this is achieved later. It is important that both eyes are affected equally, without the development of signs of suppression in either eye.

The term "amblyopia of arrest" is useful in this situation. This type of amblyopia affects both astigmatism with the rule and oblique astigmatism. Against the rule astigmatism with amblyopia is rare. Hyperopic astigmatism may with time evolve into mixed or myopic astigmatism.

Amblyopia is rare with a pure spherical bilateral refractive error. It does exist with high uncorrected bilateral hyperopia, however. This can be explained theoretically. With accommodative convergence, strabismus would develop; therefore the child prefers to see blurred but single images rather than clear and double images.

AMBLYOPIA EX ANOPSIA OR DEPRIVATION AMBLYOPIA

In recent times, there has been an effort to narrow the definition of the term "amblyopia ex anopsia" or "amblyopia of disuse." Formerly, this term encompassed every type of functional amblyopia, but it now includes only those cases in which an eye actually receives no visual impulses. Examples are dense unilateral congenital cataracts or ptosis.[107]

Such an amblyopia ex anopsia has more reference to animal experiments than it has practical significance. Experimentally, in cats and monkeys, when an eye has been deprived of light in the first month of life, atrophy in the lateral geniculate body has been found.[69] The cells in the lateral geniculate body that were innervated by the closed eye were 40% smaller than those in the open eye. Also, visual cortical cells, the majority of which normally respond to binocular stimulation, become monocular after occlusion of one eye and no longer respond to stimulation of the occluded eye. Strictly speaking, comparison of these findings with amblyopia in humans can only be allowed with amblyopia ex anopsia. In all other cases, photostimulation of the retina and cortex by light reaching the eye is possible.

BILATERAL AMBLYOPIA THROUGH DISTURBANCES OF FIXATION

Abnormal fixation is common in unilateral deep amblyopia. It may be difficult to determine whether this is based on a primary disturbance of fixation or on a central scotoma. Those rare cases of nystagmus on distance fixation that is blocked on near fixation by convergence are instructive. We had a patient who was bothered by nystagmus when attempting to shoot at a distance of 300 meters. At this distance, he could see all targets but was unable to fixate a specific one. At near gaze, he had full visual acuity and reading capacity, since the nystagmus was blocked by convergence.

Latent nystagmus has a great effect on vision. In esotropia with latent nystagmus, vision is much better when both eyes are open than when the deviating eye is occluded.

AMBLYOPIA EX ANISOMETROPIA

In anisometropic amblyopia, one eye has normal or near normal vision. The second eye has either astigmatism, or hyperopia (anisohyperopia) or myopia (anisomyopia). The same principles that apply in bilateral refractive amblyopia are also true for the amblyopic eye. The visual image on the retina is blurred and fails to stimulate full visual development. There is a significant difference, however, from bilateral amblyopia. The visual cortex gets a clear sense of the environment from the good eye. One therefore encounters the phenomenon that plays an overwhelming role in strasbismic amblyopia—namely, suppression. This is best illustrated by the following example: With monocular viewing of the Amsler grid by the amblyopic eye, primarily those lines around the central point of fixation are seen as blurred, while the peripheral lines are normal. The same is seen when the Amsler grid is presented binocularly and haploscopically in such a way that the sound eye is only shown a fixation point and peripheral borders, while an intact full grid is presented to the amblyopic eye. Under these conditions, however, a central scotoma is found that is slightly larger than the area of blurring seen on monocular presentation.

Aniseikonia (difference in image size) is frequently blamed for anisometropic amblyopia. This is not well understood. It is noteworthy, however, that children tolerate anisometropic corrections that should produce aniseikonia very well.

Amblyopia is not as severe with anisomyopia as with anisohyperopia. Differences of up to six diopters rarely cause amblyopia with myopia, since near vision is still good. With anisohyperopia and astigmatism, differences of only 1.5 diopters are enough to produce differences in vision. The greater the anisohyperopia, the more severe the amblyopia. Anisometropic amblyopia must be differentiated from microstrabismic amblyopia and from amblyopia with distinct organic findings. Treatment primarily consists of correction of the refractive anomaly. Contact lenses are needed to correct very large differences. With axial anisometropia, contact lenses increase the difference in image size, which glasses do not do. On the other hand, correction with strong-lens glasses produces a prismatic effect on lateral gaze. Monocular aphakia is the primary indication for contact lenses.

Anisometropic amblyopia slowly improves with long-term wearing of glasses. If improvement fails to occur, further measures are needed. We advise against constant full-time occlusion of the good eye, since this interrupts fusion and eventually leads to strabismus. Daily total occlusion of the sound eye for a quarter-hour to one hour should be associated with visual tasks, for example, watching television or reading. A rewarding exercise has been the finding and circling of the letter E in a block of text. One starts with larger type, then progresses to smaller type. Equally practical is mild blurring caused by glasses constantly worn in front of the good eye.

STRABISMIC AMBLYOPIA

Strabismic amblyopia is the most important type of amblyopia. Three to four percent of the entire population is strabismic. Half these patients have moderate to severe visual loss in one eye. There is no other eye disease in childhood that causes so much loss of vision and responds so well to treatment.

Is amblyopia the cause of strabismus or, vice versa, is strabismus the cause of amblyopia? Historically, this has been a significant question that often incited passion when discussed by our scientific forefathers.

The proponents of congenital amblyopia stated that esotropia developed with organic unilateral loss of vision in the first years of life (for example, with corneal opacity). Esotropia should therefore also occur with amblyopia without obvious organic changes. Cases in which amblyopia failed to respond to occlusion therapy were cited as evidence against strabismic amblyopia. This viewpoint was defended by a number of important ophthalmologists and unfortunately led to the rejection of amblyopia therapy by a large number of people for a long period of time. In fact, cases of amblyopia without strabismus and without organic changes do exist. These are often found in families in whom strabismus is prevalent. Today, we would interpret these as examples of microstrabismus.

The defenders of strabismic amblyopia were able to cite the success of occlusion therapy in support of their viewpoint. In older children, however, a very long period of occlusion led to success in only a relatively small percentage of cases.

For this reason, the concept of treating strabismic amblyopia failed to make headway in continental Europe, as it had done in England. Today we are convinced that amblyopia is the result of strabismus and not its cause.

Conversely, certain questions still exist. Is there such a thing as congenital amblyopia, and if so, how common is it? What happens with strabismic amblyopia? Is the vision of the deviating eye frozen at the level it had reached at the moment of onset of strabismus (amblyopia of arrest), or does an actual decrease in vision occur as a result of suppression (amblyopia of extinction)? How does refraction of the amblyopic eye fit in? Is there a normal emmetropization of this eye? The amblyopic eye is usually more hyperopic than the sound eye. Is this the cause or the result of amblyopia? Why is amblyopia more common with esotropia than with primary exotropia? Is the sensory disturbance or the motor disturbance the major factor in amblyopia? Clinical observations provide some direction in answering these questions. We have observed a number of infants who alternate between the two freely in the first month of life. This is the rule with congenital strabismus. At eight to twelve months, however, the strabismus becomes markedly unilateral, and deep amblyopia of the deviating eye develops. Only with intensive occlusion therapy is the child brought back to alternation. With strabismic amblyopia, one should not be dealing with simply an arrest of development but with suppression amblyopia, as was outlined previously. Congenital amblyopia should be very rare.

Suppression, which in unilateral strabismus always takes the form of zero point scotoma with foveal scotoma in the deviating eye, will become very deep and hard to reverse in a short period of time when onset is early in life. This suppression primarily affects central retinal areas, whereas the peripheral visual fields remain intact. This probably is based upon binocular rivalry and is cortical in origin. How this suppression mechanism works and where it occurs (the parastriate area, the lateral geniculate body, or the retina) is unknown.

How rapidly and intensively such a suppression can develop is shown by occlusion amblyopia. When one occludes the good eye of a small child, a very deep amblyopia sometimes develops in a brief period of time. On removing the occlusion, the child may appear virtually blind in the previously good eye. At first, he may be unable to recognize large objects and may have difficulty in orientation. The shock of the parents is understandable. Immediate reversal of occlusion usually returns normal acuity in a few days. If the situation is ignored, however, later reversal by occlusion is not always successful.

In practice, this situation is important, because one must take immediate steps while reassuring the parents. From a theoretic viewpoint, occlusion amblyopia is of great interest because it shows how variable the tendency toward amblyopia is from case to case. While one may occlude the eyes of some children for months without causing a change in fixation or significant improvement in the amblyopia, in other patients occlusion amblyopia develops with minimal full-time occlusion.

Thus, the common dictum that "visual acuity once reached can always be regained" is not totally correct. The patient's age plays a significant role in amblyopia. The intensity of suppression seems to be greater between 10 and 24 months of age. Conversely, it is during this time that suppression is most reversible; it is not reversible to the same degree after three years of age.

Since the retinal center is responsible for the exact mechanisms of fixation, the fixation mechanism is directly influenced by and dependent upon the size and intensity of the central scotoma. The fine retrograde sensory messages elicited by peripheral retinal stimuli that lead to correction of fixation into the exact foveal center are no longer adequate. The amblyopic eye has a difficulty with fixation. These fixation difficulties are naturally stronger when the strabismus is associated with disturbances in motor coordination and fixation, as is the case in congenital strabismus with latent nystagmus.

Additional clinical characteristics of strabismic amblyopia are the possible loss of central fixation, specifically the development of eccentric fixation, and typical difficulty in image separation (crowding phenomenon).[106] The hallmark of the crowding phenomenon is that single optotypes are seen better than line optotypes. That the motor aspect of separation difficulty results from fixation difficulties is illustrated in amblyopia.

With large angles of deviation, the prognosis for amblyopia treatment is considerably poorer than for microstrabismus. This is a result of motor disturbances playing an important role in large angles, whereas with microstrabismus, sensory disturbances predominate.

To understand the purely sensory disturbances associated with amblyopia, it is useful to look at those types of strabismus in which a motor disturbance is minimal. This is the case with microstrabismus. Here, too, it is more illuminating not to study deep-rooted amblyopia with dense central scotomas but to consider small decreases in vision associated with primary, previously untreated microstrabismus. Cases of anisometropia should be excluded, since anisometropia alone may cause amblyopia or may intensify amblyopia associated with microstrabismus.

Amblyopia with primary microstrabismus has various clinical characteristics. Distance vision is usually relatively good; single and row optotypes can be read up to 20/20. Difficulties develop in shooting a rifle for right-handed people who have microstrabismus in the right eye. The target is seen clearly only intermittently, finally becoming totally blurred. These patients indicate that either they are forced to shoot very rapidly or they develop into left-handed marksmen, even though they are actually right-handed. Furthermore, near acuity of the microtropic eye is considerably worse than distance acuity. The reason for this is that in a text of type, the letters are much closer to each other than are optotypes on a distance acuity chart, even with rows of optotypes. For example, on a Birkhauser distance acuity table, the optotypes for 20/20 vision are separated from each other by 25 minutes of arc, whereas on the Birkhauser reading table, 20/20 letters are separated from each other by only four to five minutes of arc. With distance vision, only one optotype is seen at a time with each eye movement. With the reading text, three or four letters are seen simultaneously. Reading difficulty can be analyzed if one uses a text in which all letters are the same size and the individual words only have four or five letters so that they can be seen with a single fixation movement.

For example, with microstrabismus of the left eye, the beginning letters are not seen clearly, whereas with right microstrabismus, it is the end letters that are unclear. These sensory defects are nicely illustrated on the Amsler grid.

In most cases with central fixation, there is no central scotoma on monocular fixation (as opposed to amblyopia ex anisometropia), but an eccentric scotoma is seen temporally. This means that in the left eye, there is a

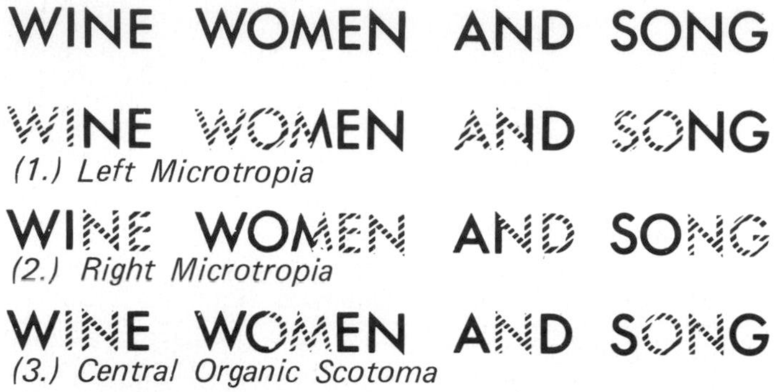

WINE WOMEN AND SONG

WINE WOMEN AND SONG
(1.) Left Microtropia

WINE WOMEN AND SONG
(2.) Right Microtropia

WINE WOMEN AND SONG
(3.) Central Organic Scotoma

Fig. 13–Reading scotoma.
1. Microstrabismus of right eye;
2. Microstrabismus of left eye; and
3. Organic central scotoma.

scotoma to the left of center, and in the right eye, to the right of fixation. The answers are more precise on the red/black Amsler grid than on a white/black grid. With a haploscopic presentation, the scotoma is somewhat larger and expands over the central point but is still more pronounced temporally. In these minimal cases, one is therefore dealing with a binocular zero point scotoma that persists monocularly as a parafoveal scotoma, causing difficulties in separation. In deeper amblyopia, such subjective answers are no longer possible, and on binocular presentation, the entire Amsler grid in front of the amblyopic eye is suppressed.

With very deep amblyopia, the fixation point scotoma blends into the central scotoma. In some cases, we may be able to plot an absolute central scotoma, on the perimeter. These sensory changes are associated with motor changes, which may accentuate such manifestations as the crowding phenomenon.

Why some cases of strabismus have deep amblyopia and others have moderate is unknown. With identical twins, one of the twins can alternate, whereas the other develops a strabismic amblyopia with eccentric fixation. Amblyopia may also vary markedly in familial cases of microstrabismus. This unpredictable nature of amblyopia, specifically suppression, is reflected in its good response to occlusion therapy, as compared with the results of treatment of anomalous retinal correspondence.

Amblyopia can be divided into severe cases (vision 0.2 [20/100] and less), moderate cases (0.2 to 0.5 [20/100–20/40]), and minimal cases (0.5 to 0.9 [20/40–20/25]). The division of amblyopia according to fixation is important — those with central fixation and those with eccentric. In the extreme case, one can diagnose a large-angle eccentric fixation from the position of the corneal reflex. It is more practical, however, to use an ophthalmoscope with a fixation mark, for example, the Visuscope, and to ask the patient to fixate the one-degree large star figure with good eye occluded. This is best done with a dim light free of red.

In addition to testing for fixation with direct opthalmoscopy, one can also use indirect ophthalmoscopy. For this purpose, one uses the Visuscope as the light source projecting the star through the indirect lens held in front of the eye. In this way, it is possible to determine fixation in very small children, even in those with constricted pupils. It is also practical in cases of severe myopia.

Fig. 14–Monocular examination on the Amsler grid. *a)* Anisometropic amblyopia: foveal scotoma; *b)* Organic central scotoma with solar retinitis; *c)* Microstrabismic amblyopia of left eye: parafoveal temporal scotoma; and *d)* Microstrabismic amblyopia of right eye: parafoveal temporal scotoma.

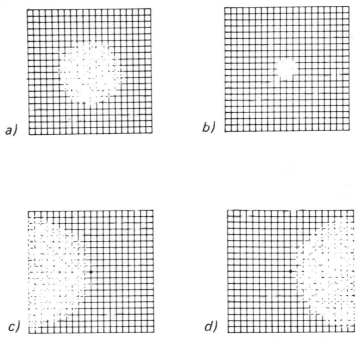

Fig. 15–Material for binocular investigation of the Amsler grid. One eye is presented a full Amsler grid, the other only the border and central point of fixation.

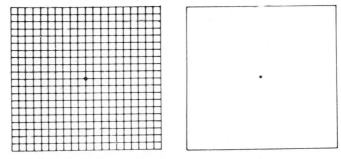

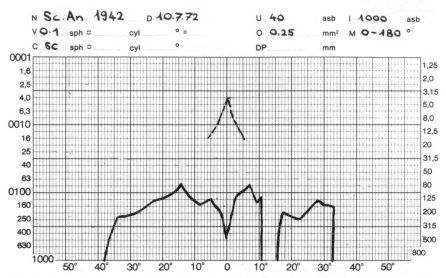

Fig. 16–Example of central scotoma determined by static perimetry in microstrabismus of the right eye with vision of 20/200.

Direct and indirect ophthalmoscopy permit a topographic localization of fixation. The terms "macula" and "paramacula" should be avoided in this connection. These regions are difficult to define, and their size varies from author to author. Duke-Elder, for example, measures the macula lutea to be 12 degrees in diameter. Klar defines the fovea as 5 degrees or 1.5 mm in diameter and recognizes it according to the wall reflex. The foveola is recognized by the foveolar reflex and has a diameter of 1.2 degrees. With central fixation, the test mark is fixated steadily within the foveola. When fixation is next to the foveola but still within the foveal reflex, parafoveolar fixation exists. Fixation in the posterior pole next to the fovea is called parafoveal. Fixation that is still within the macula and parafovea could be mistakenly labeled as paramacular. The term "paramacula" should be avoided, since the region of the macula is considerably larger than that of the fovea, and it cannot be exactly delineated. Fixation next to the disc is known as parapapillary, that in the fundus periphery as peripheral. Fixation may change according to the direction of gaze. Finally, there is also fixation that is totally unstable.

We have found it useful to make a drawing of the exact point of fixation on a fundus diagram along with the description of its characteristics: steady, unsteady, nystagmiform. One should also note the dependence of the fixation on the direction of gaze. Fundus photographs of fixation have also proven valuable in documenting organic fundus changes.

The differentiation between "eccentric fixation" and "eccentric viewing" has more theoretic than practical significance, since it cannot be made in a child and has no influence on treatment. With eccentric fixation, the patient should have the sensation that he is seeing the star as "straight ahead with his eccentric retinal area." With eccentric viewing, the subjective straight-ahead position is still at the foveola. Since there is a scotoma at the fovea, however, the patient prefers to fixate the objects with an extrafoveal point at the edge of scotoma.

The point of eccentric fixation is partially determined by the extent of the scotoma. Anomalous retinal correspondence is almost always present with eccentric fixation. It is probable that the subjective sensation of straight ahead that exists with binocular vision codetermines the point of fixation in monocular vision, especially when central scotoma is present. For this reason, in microstrabismus we almost always see that the eccentric fixation point lies on a direct connecting line between the foveola and the localizing center of the anomalous retinal correspondence.

Temporal or (paradoxic) fixation with esotropia seems to be based upon the fact that the central scotoma is not sufficiently eliminated, thereby "forcing" a motor correction. Fixation "wanders" around the scotoma, so to speak. Spontaneous temporal fixation without previous amblyopia treatment is rare.

Usually, only one eye has eccentric fixation. Occasionally, however, one can show eccentric fixation in both eyes. With congenital strabismus in very small children, it is not uncommon for the star to be fixated nasal to the foveola in each eye; at the same time, a jerky nystagmus toward the foveola is present. With time, fixation moves toward the foveola. In cases with gaze paresis, a bilateral eccentric fixation may also be present. For example, in gaze paresis to the right, the right eye may have a nasal eccentric fixation, the

Fig. 17–Fixation types: 1, central fixations, 2, parafoveolar fixation, 3, parafoveal fixation, 5 & 6, peripheral fixation, and 4, parapapillary fixation.

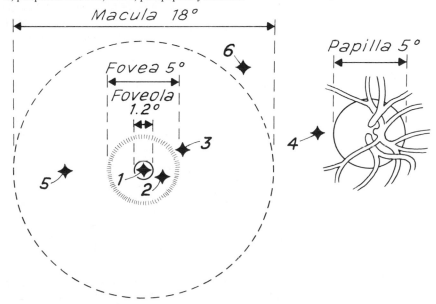

left eye a temporal eccentric fixation. The same is true for patients with homonymous hemianopsia. With a left hemianopic central scotoma, there is nasal eccentric fixation in the right eye, and a temporal eccentric fixation in the left eye. With bilateral organic macula damage or central scotoma due to optic atrophy, eccentric fixation occurs over the fovea bilaterally.

The concepts of eccentric fixation and retinal correspondence are often confused. Anomalous retinal correspondence is a binocular phenomenon; eccentric fixation is a monocular phenomenon. Anomalous retinal correspondence can occur with both alternating and monocular strabismus, while fixation can be central or eccentric. Eccentric fixation occurs almost exclusively with anomalous retinal correspondence. Amblyopia with eccentric fixation responds to therapy, whereas anomalous retinal correspondence is more resistant to therapy.

Treatment of amblyopia will be dealt with in greater detail in Chapter 4. The age at which therapy is begun is of greatest prognostic significance. The earlier it is instituted, the better the results. Therefore, the diagnosis must be established as early as possible. This is easy with cosmetically obvious monocular strabismus. A small child with microstrabismus is more difficult to diagnose. The possibility that microstrabismus is present is increased in cases of intermittent monocular strabismus, as it is with siblings of strabismics. Careful stereopsis testing — for example, with the Lang stereo test, fixation testing, and refraction — must be done in these patients.

ACCOMMODATION AND CONVERGENCE

Throughout life, close objects receive more attention and interest than those at a distance. This is particularly true in early childhood, when a child is most concerned with the environment within his reach. This is also true for stereopsis, which functions primarily within the distance of one's reach, out to 10 meters.

ACCOMMODATION

In order to see a nearby object clearly, the eye must accommodate. Equally strong impulses reach the ciliary muscles via parasympathetic fibers of the ocular motor nerve. The ciliary muscle contracts through parasympathetic innervation. Sympathetic innervation plays a role in relaxation.

As the ciliary muscle contracts, the zonular fibers relax. Because of its elasticity, the lens takes on a more spheric form, thereby increasing accommodation. Accommodation is measured in diopters. In viewing an object at infinity, the eye needs no accommodation. If the object is at a distance of one meter, one diopter of accommodation must be used in order to see it clearly. At a distance of 50 centimeters, two diopters of accommodation is needed, at 33 centimeters three diopters is needed, and so forth.

Accommodation in diopters is the inverse of the distance to the object in meters. According to the formula:

$$\text{Accommodations in D} = \frac{1}{\text{object distance in meters}}$$

The near point of accommodation is that point at which, with maximal accommodation, one can still see clearly. The range between distance and near point of accommodation is known as the accommodative range. In the course of life, the elasticity of the lens decreases and therewith the range of accommodation, leading to presbyopia. Two further processes are linked to accommodation: constriction of the pupil and convergence of the two eyes.

CONVERGENCE

The two eyes must converge in order to see a near object as a single image. This means that the visual line of both eyes should intersect at the point of fixation. The angle formed by these two visual lines is known as the convergence angle. The point at which these two visual lines intersect with maximal convergence is the near point of convergence. The angle of convergence is dependent upon the distance to the fixated object and the interpupillary distance. The nearer the object of fixation and the greater the interpupillary distance, the more convergence is required, and the larger is the convergence angle (Fig. 18).

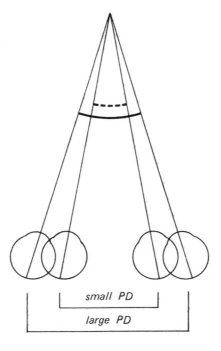

Fig. 18–Relationship between the angle of convergence and the interpupillary distance.

Convergence is not evoked by a single stimulus, but by a variety of inducing mechanisms and factors. Voluntary convergence makes it possible to converge at will — for example, at the tip of one's nose. This convergence can be practiced.

Proximal convergence is induced by the psychic sensation of an object being nearby. This plays a role in so-called "instrument convergence." Although instruments such as binoculars or a synoptophore are set for distance, when brought close to the eye they will elicit a convergence movement.

Fusional convergence is an involuntary movement to see objects that lie very close to each other as binocular and single.

Tonic convergence is the baseline innervation of convergence. It is particularly prominent in small children but decreases over the years. It is dependent upon a number of factors, including the emotional state (increase in convergence with embarrassment and anger). Accommodative convergence is convergence that is linked with accommodative effort. It can be elicited by wearing concave lenses in front of the eyes for distance viewing. If a –3.00 diopter glass is placed in front of one eye of a person with normal binocular vision while the other eye is occluded, and that person is asked to fixate on an object at a short distance, three diopters of accommodation are required to see the object clearly. At the same time, the covered eye converges a set amount. The same occurs if an object is brought up to 33 centimeters. In this case, three diopters of accommodation are required, to which is linked an amount of convergence that differs for each individual. When this is excessive or insufficient, adjustment is made in fusion.

Since the angle of convergence depends upon the interpupillary distance, the angle of convergence must be calculated trigonometrically for each individual in order to be expressed in degrees or prism diopters.

A universal measure of convergence therefore is the meter angle, analogous to diopters as the unit of measurement for accommodation. If a fixation object is at a distance of one meter, an emmetrope must accommodate one diopter and at the same time converge a one-meter angle in order to see the object clearly and binocularly singly. For an object at a distance of 50 centimeters, accommodation is two diopters and convergence is two meter angles; at a distance of 33 centimeters, three diopters of accommodation and a three-meter angle of convergence are required.

The relationship of accommodation to convergence can be represented graphically with a coordinate system. On the horizontal abscissa, convergence is represented in meter angles, and on the vertical ordinate, accommodation appears in diopters. The integration of accommodation and convergence results in the convergence or Donders' line (Fig. 19).

Convergence and divergence can be varied slightly without changing accommodation. This is known as relative range of convergence and is shown in Fig. 20 for an accommodation of three diopters. Accommodation can vary when the angle of convergence is held steady. This is shown in Fig. 21 for a convergence of two-meter angles. This is known as the relative range of accommodation.

Accommodation of all these ranges can be represented in a graph. On each side of the convergence line, an area is indicated in which fusion occurs.

Accommodative convergence plays a large role in heterophoria and strabismus. It can be measured with the alternate prism cover test, by which fusion is suspended. The deviation is measured for distance and near gaze. Accommodation must be controlled. At near gaze, a small optotype should be fixated and seen clearly. Existing refractive errors must therefore be fully corrected. By measuring convergence at varying distances, proximal convergence is not released.

The other possibility is always to fixate distance objects and stimulate accommodation by use of minus lenses, or to fixate a near object and to relax the accommodation by use of plus lenses.

The results can be recorded on the coordinate system. For this, the meter angle has to be calculated in prism diopters or degrees.

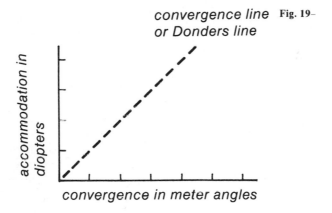

convergence line Fig. 19–
or Donders line

accommodation in diopters

convergence in meter angles

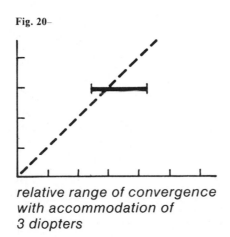

Fig. 20–

relative range of convergence
with accommodation of
3 diopters

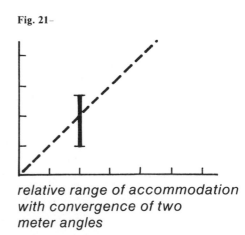

Fig. 21–

relative range of accommodation
with convergence of two
meter angles

One prism diopter deviates a beam of light from a one-meter distance by one centimeter. With an interpupillary distance of six centimeters, both eyes must converge six prism diopters when the object is at a distance of one meter. At 33 centimeters, the convergence is three times greater. In other words, with an interpupillary distance of six centimeters, convergence equals 18 prism diopters. One can therefore state the following formula:

Convergence angle in diopters = accommodation (in diopters) × the
pupillary distance (in centimeters)

By this formula, one meter angle of convergence in diopters equals the interpupillary distance in centimeters.

For a pupillary distance of six centimeters, one meter angle equals six diopters; two meter angles equal 12 diopters. For an interpupillary distance of five centimeters, five meter angles equal five diopters; two meter angles equal 10 diopters.

Recalculating meter angles in degrees using the 360 degrees of the circle is complicated. The formula reads:

$$\text{tang } 1/2 \text{ Convergence angle} = \frac{1/2PD}{\text{object distance}}$$

The tangent of half the angle of convergence is equal to half the pupillary distance divided by the distance to the object. To convert degrees into prism

Fig. 22–Enlargement of Donders' scheme. (The value for interpupillary distance is 60 mm; at a PD of 65 mm, one meter angle would equal 65 diopters.)

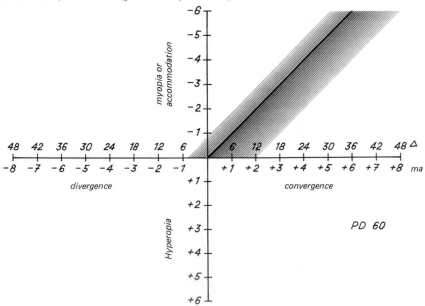

diopters: Four degrees equal seven prism diopters. Frequently, one degree is converted into two prism diopters. This is a rough approximation. One (1) degree is 1.745 prism diopters, or one (1) prism diopter is 0.57 degrees. Since prism diopters represent a linear measurement, one should not add them. It is best to convert all values with a via tangents into arc degrees using a calculator.

When the clinically obtained values are entered into the formulas, the slope of the convergence line reflects the relationship between accommodation and convergence. With a flat sloping convergence line, more convergence than accommodation is exerted; there is a convergence excess (Fig. 23). With a steep slope of the convergence line, less convergence is exerted than accommodation, and there is a convergence insufficiency (Fig. 24). The term "divergence excess" is to be avoided, since we do not believe that divergence is an active process. Instead, we feel that one is dealing with a convergence excess with a position of rest in divergence.

During growth, there is an increase in the pupillary distance, increasing the slope of the convergence line. This means that there is a decrease in convergence excess.

In the English-speaking literature, the relationship of accommodative convergence to accommodation is called the AC/A ratio. A high AC/A ratio implies excessive convergence. With a low AC/A ratio, little convergence is produced in relationship to accommodation, equivalent to a weakness in convergence. In order to talk about an increased AC/A ratio or convergence

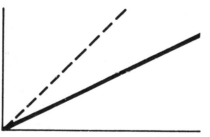

Figs. 23 and 24–Slope of the convergence line with convergence excess and convergence insufficiency.

convergence excess, high AC/A ratio

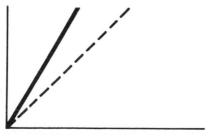

convergence insufficiency, low AC/A ratio

excess, the angle at near gaze should be more than 10 prism diopters greater than that for distance. This must be tested with accommodation controlled.

Several methods can be used to test for the accommodation/convergence relationship. With the heterophoria method, the alternate cover test is done for distance, with full correction of any refractive errors. Subsequently, with accommodation controlled, the same is done at a distance of 33 or 50 centimeters. The difference between the near and distance heterophoria divided by the amount of accommodation plus the interpupillary distance gives the AC/A ratio.

In the gradient method, examination is done at the same distance but with either concave or convex lenses in place. For example, while viewing a test target at 5 meters, a concave lens of –1.50, 2.00, or 3.00 diopters is used. On near testing at 33 centimeters, the deviation is measured without correction but with +1.00, +2.00, or +3.00 diopter lenses in place.

For example, if with optical correction a patient is orthophoric at distance but with a –3.00 diopter lens shows an esophoria of 12 diopters, each diopter of accommodation has elicited four diopters of convergence. The AC/A ratio is then four to one.

The average AC/A ratio in adults is 3.50 diopters of accommodative convergence for each diopter of accommodation. It differs from person to person and is dependent on the testing methods employed.

Further discussions about accommodative convergence can be found in the chapters on heterophoria and types of strabismus.

HEREDITY OF STRABISMUS

Hippocrates stated that "strabismics beget strabismics." Reports about the familial occurrence of strabismus give a probability of up to 50%. Since the incidence of strabismus in the general population is 4%, one should easily find several cases of strabismus in any study of a large family. Statements about the familial incidence are therefore not very useful unless the number of family members and generations examined is specifically spelled out.

As previously mentioned, strabismus is not a uniform entity. There are various types of strabismus, as well as many factors that either singly or in concert can lead to strabismus. Strabismus has a multifactorial etiology. It is useful to attempt to delineate these hereditary factors and conditions by trying to separate them out in the family history if possible.

Primary microstrabismus has been shown by Richter and us to have a hereditary tendency.[94] This inherited tendency is independent of the actual or refractive error and encompasses only the anomalous retinal correspondence. Amblyopia may be minimal or very severe.[1,22,86]

Esophoria can be inherited. It is not uncommon to find a clustering of esophoria patients in one family. Exophoria is also frequently familial. In this situation, one thinks about those families in whom individuals with large interpupillary distances and intermittent divergence strabismus are found. "A" and "V" patterns can also be hereditary, as can cocontraction syndromes. Refractive errors have distinctly hereditary factors, whether we deal with myopia, hyperopia, astigmatism, or anisometropia. Convergence excess or high AC/A ratio often appears to be inherited.

The combination of one or more of such hereditary predispositions determines the type of strabismus in individual cases. It is therefore useful to pay attention to the hereditary relationships in strabismus, both from a theoretical and practical viewpoint.

In our experience, congenital strabismus has little tendency to be hereditary. External factors such as prematurity and birth trauma seem to play an important role. Of interest are studies on identical twins in whom different types of strabismus can occur.

2

DIAGNOSIS

The clinical history should be taken at the beginning of the first visit. During this time, one can observe the patient's overall behavior, head position, ocular alignment, and so forth.

As in all other areas of medicine, the clinical history is extremely valuable in strabismus. It is, so to speak, half the examination. The ability to ask the right questions and therefore elicit more valuable answers increases the understanding the examiner has of his subject material.

Similarly, the more recent the onset of the strabismus, the more reliable and exact the answer. For example, adult strabismics usually are vague about the time of onset of their strabismus if it dates back to early childhood. When examining small children, one can often obtain precise information from the parents about the onset of the strabismus and its characteristics.

CLINICAL HISTORY OF THE STRABISMUS

When did the child's eyes begin to cross? The point in time of the onset of strabismus is of great differential diagnostic and prognostic value. If a child is said to have had strabismus since birth, one should remember that intermittent convergence spasms do occur in infants, and that this may not be of particular significance. Only constant strabismus in the first few months of life is significant. Similarly, a pseudostrabismus due to epicanthal folds may confuse the history. It is useful to separate when the strabismus "really" developed from when it "got worse."

How did the strabismus begin? Was it of sudden onset or gradually increasing? Was the angle of deviation constant, alternating, or intermittent? Is it related to fatigue or emotions? Are the eyes ever straight? Is the deviation worse in the morning (essential paresis) or in the evening (accommodative), or greater at near gaze (convergence excess)?

Which eye deviates? Always the same or alternating? With unilateral slowly increasing strabismus, one should think of a decompensating microstrabismus. Did the patient close one eye with the onset of the strabismus (diplopia with acute late onset strabismus and normal sensory relationships), or does he close one eye in bright light or outside in the sun (intermittent exotropia)?

Is there a head tilt (congenital strabismus or paresis)? In doubtful cases, old photographs are useful.

What triggered the strabismus: measles, pertussis, psychologic trauma, or some other cause? A relationship with a previous illness is remembered less frequently by the parents the more recent the clinical onset. In fact, several years after the onset of strabismus, its cause may be related by the patient or his parents to be an illness that actually occurred months after the true onset. What treatment has been instituted since the onset of the strabismus — atropinization, occlusion, glasses, orthoptics, surgery? With what results?

Prenatal and postnatal factors of interest include infectious diseases, trauma, prematurity, and birth weight. Was the child asphyxiated? Was there an Rh factor incompatibility with kernicterus? What was the Apgar score? What childhood illnesses have occurred? Is development normal? Are there signs of brain damage?

Postnatal development of the child can be divided into the following time periods:

1. the *newborn* period, during the first three weeks of life.

2. *infancy*, from the third week to the first year of life.

3. the *small child* or *toddler*, from one to six years of age.

4. *school age*, from six to fifteen years. This period includes puberty.

FAMILY HISTORY

A sketch of the family tree belongs in each medical record for rapid orientation of subsequent consultants. Do other family members have strabismus? If so, then the various types of strabismus and their course should be recorded. Do other family members have amblyopia (microstrabismus or anisometropic amblyopia)? We have made it a rule to look for microstrabismus in parents and siblings using the Lang-Stereo test for rapid screening.

INSPECTION

The most obvious finding in marked strabismus is the cosmetic deviation. This represents a true handicap to the patient. The untrained observer may notice only that "something is not right with the eyes" but is unable to specify whether an eye deviates in or out. It takes particular training to gain as much information as possible for such a simple inspection.

At the time of taking the history, one looks for an abnormal head position. The head may turn around three axes (Fig. 25):

— *vertical:* the face is turned to the right or left;

— *transversal:* the chain is elevated or depressed;

— *sagittal:* the head is tilted either to the right or to the left shoulder.

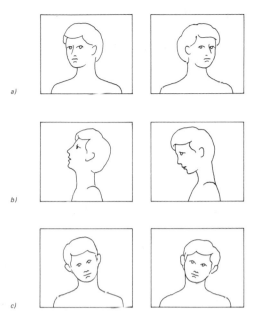

a)

b)

c)

Fig. 25–Abnormal head positions.
a) Face turn,
b) Chin elevation and depression,
c) Head tilt to the shoulder.

One must differentiate between muscular or ocular tilt and torticollis. Muscular torticollis is due to fibrosis of the sternocleidomastoid muscle. The head is tilted toward the involved side. Active and passive tilt toward the other side is limited. On palpation, one can feel the stiffness of the involved muscle. Such a head tilt leads to asymmetry of the face. The side of the face on the side of the tilt is smaller and underdeveloped. Orthopedic treatment is indicated in the first year of life. Patients should be referred to orthopedic surgeons. Deformation of the vertebrae can lead to a similar abnormal head position.

Ocular torticollis does not lead to facial asymmetry because the abnormal position does not persist in sleep. In eye muscle paresis, the head is turned in such a way that the paretic muscle is out of its field of action. This is to avoid diplopia. For example, with paresis of the right medial rectus the face is turned left, the eyes right. With nystagmus, the head position is that in which the amplitude of nystagmus is least (position of rest, null point). With astigmatism or cylindric corrections, the head may be held abnormally in order to achieve clearer vision.

In the "A" and "V" syndromes, the chin may be depressed or elevated to achieve that position of gaze which allows singular binocular vision. With congenital strabismus, there is often a head tilt, usually to one shoulder or with a face turn.

Not only the ocular position but also the configuration of the lids plays a large role in strabismus. Mongoloid slants are observed with "A" patterns, antimongoloid slants with "V" patterns.

Pseudostrabismus is important. Epicanthal folds can simulate esotropia, since the nasal sclera is less exposed than the temporal one. On right or left gaze, the sclera may disappear entirely behind the epicanthal fold, simulating esotropia of the adducted eye. This impression may be so pronounced that it is difficult to persuade the parents that strabismus is not present, and no therapy is needed. Diagnosis of the true eye position is made by observing the corneal light reflexes: If both are equally positioned slightly nasal to the pupillary center, a true strabismus is probably not present. Often, one can confirm this impression by use of the alternate cover test, even in small children. The placing of base-out prisms before one eye may evoke a fusional movement, indicating normal binocular vision. The corneal light reflexes are best seen in and evaluated by coaxial illumination, as through a bright direct ophthalmoscope. At the same time, equality of the observed red fundus reflex indicates ocular alignment and no significant anisometropia or unilateral media opacities, while inequality of the red fundus reflex may indicate these conditions. Observation of the red fundus reflex with an ophthalmoscope also gives useful orientation about the refraction. With hyperopia or with a myopia of up to 2.50 diopters, the upper pupillary half is brighter. With myopia of two diopters and greater, the lower pupillary half appears brighter.

In pseudostrabismus, one often learns from the history that the child has had strabismus "since birth," and that it worsens with fatigue and on sideward gaze. It is our experience that in this situation, one cannot simply tell the parents "there is no strabismus." Rather, one must explain the situation carefully: This is a pseudostrabismus that does not require therapy. Otherwise, the parents will shop from doctor to doctor until the child becomes the proud possessor of a pair of glasses or possibly has to undergo occlusion therapy! The Lang stereo test has shown itself to be ideal for the diagnosis of pseudostrabismus even in small children, thereby reassuring the parents.

Esotropia may on occasion be simulated in adults with slightly protuberant eyes if exposure of the temporal sclera is greater and the lower lid is slightly depressed temporally. The same impression is evoked when the medial portion of the upper lid is lower. Similarly, divergence strabismus may be simulated when the nasal lid area is slightly enlarged.

A small interpupillary distance may simulate esotropia, whereas a larger interpupillary distance gives the impression of exotropia.

Strabismus may also be simulated by a nasal or temporal kappa angle. The optical axis, that is, the line connecting fovea to fixation object, rarely goes through the pupillary center. In hyperopic eyes it is often displaced nasally, in myopic eyes temporally. Here, too, one can make the diagnosis according to the corneal reflex (Hirschberg). The examiner uses a muscle light held beneath his dominant eye and observes the corneal light reflex in the pupil. The same light reflex viewed coaxially through the ophthalmoscope against the red background of the fundus reflex is easier to evaluate than it is against a dark background with noncoaxial illumination. The nasally displaced or

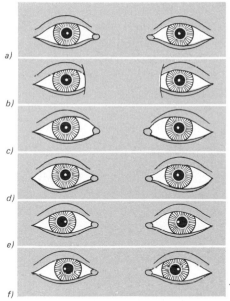

Fig. 26–
a) Straight eyes;
b) Pseudoesotropia simulated by epicanthal folds;
c) Pseudoexotropia simulated by wide nasal lid fissures;
d) Pseudoesotropia simulated by wide temporal lid fissures;
e) Pseudoexotropia simulated by a positive (nasal) kappa angle (observed position of corneal light reflex); and
f) Pseudoesotropia simulated by negative (temporal) kappa angle.

positive kappa angle simulates divergent strabismus: a temporally displaced or negative kappa angle simulates convergent strabismus. The visual axis of the eye is often called the "line of sight" or "face line."

The kappa angle is that angle formed by the visual axis and a line through the center of the pupil. One often speaks of an alpha angle, which is the angle between the visual axis and the optical axis, and/or a gamma angle, formed by the optical axis and the line connecting the center of rotation of the eye with the object of fixation (fixation axis). The lambda angle is similar to the kappa angle but refers to the center of the entrance pupil. This apparent pupil lies slightly anterior to the true pupil.[81] A nasal or positive kappa angle is fairly common, especially with hyperopia. A temporally displaced or negative angle is more rare and appears with severe myopia.

The impression of the angle of deviation is given primarily by the relationship between temporal and nasal scleral triangles. Approximation of the angle of deviation is possible by observation of the position of the corneal light reflex, as per Hirschberg. If the corneal reflex of the deviating eye is at the pupillary margin, the angle is approximately 15 degrees. If it is in the center between pupil and limbus, it is about 20 degrees, and if at the limbus, 45 degrees. The kappa angle must be included in the calculation. Every millimeter on the cornea is a deviation of about eight degrees.[63] Paliaga and coworkers have shown that this value is greater with adduction than with abduction, and that the rotation decreases in the periphery. Whereas a shift of one millimeter in the corneal center represents an angle of seven to eight degrees at the corneal periphery, this represents a rotation of only five to six degrees.[105] With very dark pupils, the pupillary margin may be difficult to see, even with a good flashlight. Examination through the retinoscope or with an ophthalmoscope outlines the pupil and allows better evaluation of the corneal reflex against the red fundus reflex. At times, the yellow of the disc may be visible in one eye, indicating a deviation of about 15 degrees onto the optic disc (blind spot mechanism of Swan). It has proven useful to draw the corneal light reflex schematically. One can then see the degree of deviation from a glance at the drawing.

Observation of the corneal reflex on the Maddox scale is of great value in estimation of the angle of deviation, especially with unilateral amblyopia with eccentric fixation. The patient sits at a distance of one meter in front of the tangent scale, first fixating the central light. With his back to the scale, sitting directly beneath the fixation light, the observer notes the corneal reflex of the patient. The patient then follows the index finger of the examiner, who moves it along the scale until the corneal reflex in the nonfixing eye is in the center of the pupil. The number on the scale to which the index finger is pointing at that time indicates the angle of deviation (Fig. 28). The kappa angle must be considered.

Similar determination of the angle of deviation is possible at the arc perimeter. The chin of the patient is placed so that the deviated eye is centered on the perimeter. With the good eye, the patient fixates straight ahead over the arc perimeter. The examiner moves a light along the arc of the perimeter until this light reflex appears in the center of the pupil of the deviating eye. The point on the perimeter where this occurs gives the angle of deviation.

Further determination of the angle of deviation, especially with high degrees of amblyopia, can be achieved by centering the corneal reflex by means of prisms (Krimsky). Prisms are placed in front of the fixing eye, forcing it to deviate until the corneal reflex appears in the center of the pupil of the nonfixing eye.

It is useful to document the angle of deviation with photographs. With concomitant strabismus, the primary position suffices; with paretic strabismus, one should document the strabismus in different positions of gaze. In the primary position, the patient should look directly at the camera lens, with the flash mounted vertically above it. In this way, one can precisely determine the position of the first Purkinje reflex. A refinement of this photographic method, especially with small angles, occurs through observation of the fourth Purkinje reflex, namely that from the posterior lens surface.[94] This is considerably smaller and weaker than the reflex from the corneal surface. It lies at the pupillary plane. One must therefore carefully center on the limbus. The fourth Purkinje image appears below and somewhat temporal to the first Purkinje image, with a nasal kappa angle. By comparing the connecting line between the first and fourth image of each eye, one can measure angles of two to five degrees.

One should also observe whether the angle of deviation is constant or varies. Is the same eye always deviated, or is there spontaneous alternation?

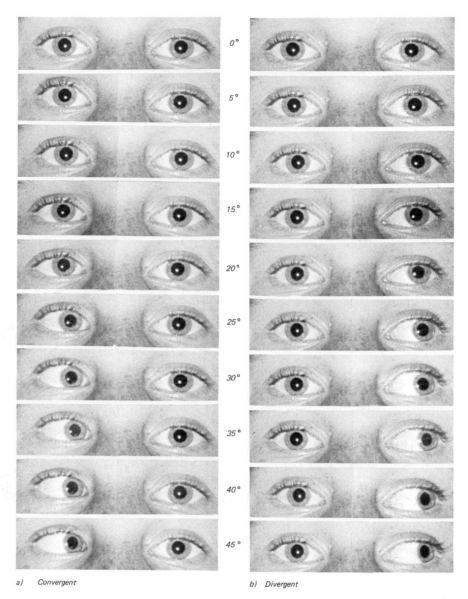

	0°
	5°
	10°
	15°
	20°
	25°
	30°
	35°
	40°
	45°

a)   *Convergent*   b)   *Divergent*

Fig. 27–*a*) Esotropia, *b*) Exotropia. Photomontage of various angles of deviation. One should observe the existence of a positive kappa angle. With abduction and in the corneal periphery, the reflex is shifted more.

Finally, is nystagmus present or not?

Similarly, one should determine eye movements. To do this, the patient is asked to look in the direction of the nine cardinal positions of gaze while following a toy or fixation light. One decides if excursion in all directions is equal and properly carried out. Does one eye deviate up or down in right or

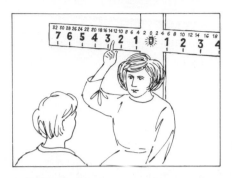

Fig. 28–Determination of the angle of strabismus by means of the corneal light reflex at the Maddox cross.

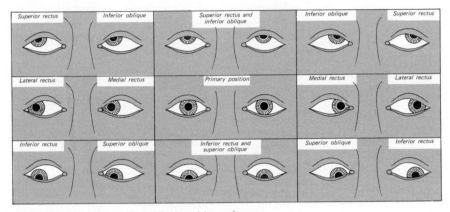

Fig. 29–The nine diagnostic cardinal positions of gaze.

left gaze? Does the angle of deviation remain constant or is it variable? The excursions can be measured at the perimeter.

Infants may occasionally be more easily examined when they are lying down. If one wants to determine upgaze, one should lay them on their stomach. One should also look for the setting sun sign in infants, where both eyes are deviated downward.

Testing for convergence is best done with a small fixation object. One determines if it occurs normally, or if convergence deficit or convergence excess is present.

GENERAL OPHTHALMIC EXAMINATION FOR VISION TESTING

Exact visual acuity testing using tumbling E's can often be carried out in intelligent children by three years of age. It is helpful for the mother or orthoptist to have previously taught the "E game" to the child so that he is able to indicate the position of the E by holding his fingers in the same direction. Besides the tumbling E's, there are a number of visual acuity charts developed specifically for children. The Landolt's rings are very well adapted for near vision testing, by use of such questions as "where can a mouse leave the circle?"

If measurement of visual acuity is not possible, one can estimate acuity. If spontaneous alternating strabismus is present, vision is equal in both eyes. With monocular strabismus, one must be concerned about amblyopia. On covering the fixing eye, if the deviating eye picks up fixation and holds it, even after the cover is removed, amblyopia is unlikely. If fixation is not maintained after removing the cover, amblyopia should be suspected. One can get a reasonable estimation whether central fixation or gross eccentric fixation is present by watching the eye movements of the deviating eye as it picks up fixation. If on covering the fixing eye, the child attempts to escape from the cover and becomes restless, but does not do this when the deviating eye is covered, amblyopia is probable. When amblyopia is suspected, ophthalmoscopic testing for fixation should be done. In small children, one determines the pupillary reflex to light, the child's reaction to a dazzling bright light, and following movements.

Refraction is determined with retinoscopy or with a refractometer after one-half to one per cent atropine drops or ointment has been instilled three times a day for three days. Retinoscopy is difficult in small children because the lens or retinoscopy bars placed in front of the eye disturb them.

Ideally, one should carry out atropine retinoscopy in every strabismic child once a year. If one is forced to use other cycloplegic drugs, the best are homatropine and Cyclogyl. Retinoscopy should be performed 20 to 30 minutes after administration.

Values obtained with cycloplegia should always be rechecked with retinoscopy with miosis. Retinoscopy is easier in miosis because the disturbing edge phenomena fall away. With small children who will not allow trial lenses to be put in front of them, one can use the previously mentioned pupillary light reflex findings to estimate the refraction. (See the section on sensory testing for evaluation of binocular cooperation.)

A complete eye examination with slit lamp and ophthalmoscope will detect corneal opacities, macular lesions, or other organic causes responsible for amblyopia or strabismus. One should look for surgical scars from previous strabismus operations and record them.

COVER–UNCOVER TEST

The cover test is the most important diagnostic test in daily ocular motility practice. One covers one eye of the patient and observes the resultant eye movements. There are various modifications of the cover test, which should be selected according to the needs in each individual case. The examination is simple, quick, and does not require a large instrumentarium. It can be carried out in small children. Since one is dealing with objectively visible eye movements, the results are independent of subjective answers and not questionable.

To get the most out of this source of information requires practice and knowledge. It is necessary to be familiar with all the details of execution and the various possible results of the test. One only sees what one understands.

A prerequisite is that the patient fixates on an object for at least a brief period of time. With adults and older children, one should routinely do the cover test for both near and distant fixation. For distance, it is best to fixate the light on the Maddox cross at five to six meters. It is too much to ask small children to fix on a simple light. For many years, therefore, we have used a special fixation device that has proven extremely useful. In a box we have a fixation light, and in front of this light there is a rotating disc with red, green, yellow, blue, and orange filters. The light therefore changes its color constantly. At the same time, a music box begins to play when the fixation light is turned on. In this way, we arouse the attention of the child. Cartoons and animated animals serve similar purposes.

The measured results at near gaze will differ with the size of the test object used. The angle of deviation in convergent strabismus will increase when a small optotype is fixated (thereby stimulating accommodation) more than when a light source is used.

For near fixation, we use a small vertical stick on which a number of pictures appear one above the other; for example, a car, a clock, a bear, a sail boat, a cat, and so forth. This variety helps the small child maintain fixation during the cover test. Children who either cannot or will not name the objects are allowed simply to point at them. On the back of the fixation bar are vertical rows of numbers for testing adults. We have applied the same pictures to a small cube on a stick, which can then be rotated to present the different pictures to the child. The various pictures are shown only one at a time. This is an advantage in examining very small children.

The cover test is done using the outstretched hand of the examiner or an occluder. We prefer the occluder because with it one can rapidly and precisely cover and uncover for better observation.

With small children and infants, the cover test is possible only at near gaze. We recommend a light such as the muscle light used for testing the corneal light reflex, held at 60 centimeters. With infants, one cannot use an occluder, since this is immediately fixated by the child. It is best to rest one's hand on the head of the child, using the thumb for occlusion. Small, rapidly moving loud toys, for example, a pinwheel that produces sparks, are excellent fixation objects. Examination must be done in an unhurried manner in order not to frighten the child. Whispering or whistling will evoke attention. In this way, the child considers the examination a game of peek-a-boo.

There are three types of cover test. They are used differently according to the case and the information desired.

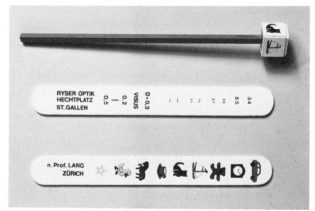

Fig. 30–Fixation stick and cube.

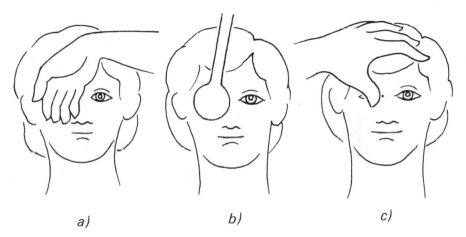

Fig. 31–Occlusion. *a*) With the hand; *b*) with occluder; and *c*) with thumb.

UNILATERAL COVER TEST

For example, the observer covers the right eye while observing the behavior of the left eye. If the left eye makes a fixation movement, this indicates that it was not previously directed at the object of fixation and that there was manifest strabismus.

If the left eye fails to move, one should remove the cover, leaving both eyes free for a few moments. One then covers the left eye while observing the behavior of the right eye. If this eye makes a fixation movement, right manifest strabismus is present.

It helps if one knows the fixating or preferred eye ahead of time. This can be determined by asking the patient to block the examiner's nose out of his line of vision with his index finger. The subject will always put his index finger in front of the fixing or dominant eye. The same can be achieved by looking through a hole in a piece of cardboard. The opening is always held in front of the dominant eye.

Further confirmation of the fixing or dominant eye is obtained by "near point of convergence" testing. The eye that deviates first is nondominant. With small children, if one is not certain which eye is fixing, the examiner can hold a vertical prism in front of one eye to see if a refixation movement occurs. The cover-uncover test is particularly indicated in determining whether strabismus is or is not present, as with pseudostrabismus and microstrabismus. With very careful observation, it is possible to see movements as small as one to two degrees, assuming that there is central fixation and no nystagmus.

If with the cover test nystagmus suddenly develops, one is dealing with latent nystagmus. This occurs commonly in congenital esotropia.

Following surgery, the cover-uncover test is an important tool for the prescription of glasses or the use of prisms to determine whether or not the eyes are straight or a residual angle is present.

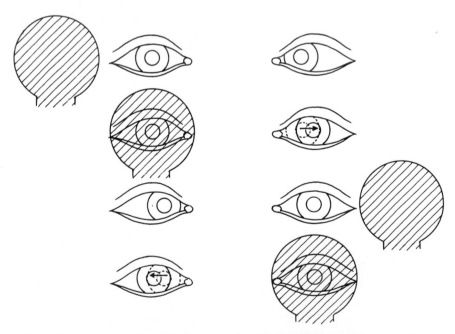

Fig. 32–The monocular cover/uncover test. At first, the right eye is covered and the left eye is observed for any shift in fixation. After leaving both eyes open for a short period, the left eye is covered and the right eye is observed for any shift in fixation.

With the alternate cover test, the eyes are alternately covered and uncovered in rapid sequence without allowing both eyes to be uncovered simultaneously. This disrupts fusion. The latent deviation becomes manifest; or with a manifest deviation, the angle may increase to that of the motor position of rest.

If with the unilateral cover–uncover test there is no strabismus, but the alternate cover test shows refixation movements, then heterophoria is present. If movement is seen with the unilateral cover–uncover test, then the alternate cover test will also show a refixation movement. If this refixation movement is equal in amplitude with both tests, then the manifest angle of deviation coincides with the fusion-free position of rest.

Often with manifest strabismus, however, the angle measured with the alternate cover test increases. This maximal angle represents a fusion-free motor position of rest. The manifest smaller deviation in a sense represents the sensory position of rest, as seen for example with anomalous retinal correspondence. This difference is important, since surgery attempts to correct the fusion-free maximal deviation measured with the alternate cover test.

With the alternate cover test, the smallest deviation that can be measured is one to two degrees. Smaller refixation movements may be observed by the patient if he notices small shifts in the fixation light with the alternate cover test. This is known as the parallax test.

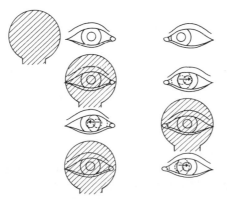

Fig. 33–Alternate cover test. The eyes are covered then uncovered one after the other in sequence while observing the refixation movements of the recently uncovered eye.

THE UNCOVER TEST

Along with the cover test, one can observe the behavior of the just-uncovered eye (uncover test). With both eyes now open, various possibilities exist:

1. The uncovered eye continues in its deviated position.

2. It picks up fixation while the other eye becomes strabismic. In this case, amblyopia should be suspected.

3. It makes a fusional movement. The previously fixing eye does not move, while the recently uncovered eye approaches a parallel position. In this case, one is dealing with heterophoria with fusional movements.

In certain cases, such as microstrabismus, fusional movement leads not to parallelism but to a smaller angle. This can be shown by immediately covering the fixing eye.

For example, the monocular cover–uncover test detects left esotropia of three degrees, which increases on the alternate cover test to six degrees. After uncovering the left eye (both eyes are now open), this eye makes a fusional divergence movement from the six degree esotropia position but does not reach parallelism. Instead, it stops at three degrees. This can be shown by means of a unilateral cover test of the right eye at that point. The cover test, therefore, gives information about the function of the fusion mechanism, even with anomalous retinal correspondence.

The cover test is also important with exodeviations. It allows differentiation between intermittent and constant divergence strabismus.

In some cases, it is useful to observe not only the uncovered eye but also the covered one. In this way, one may find alternating sursumduction, in which the covered eye deviates upward beneath the cover and comes down upon being uncovered.

With practice, one is able to judge quite accurately the size of refixation movements. To learn this, one can ask patients to fixate first on the central light and then on the number four on the Maddox scale, providing a shift of four degrees. Similarly, one can use larger or smaller angles.

In the English-speaking literature, in the cover–uncover test, covering the eye is immediately followed by uncovering it. We prefer to do this in separate steps, however.

THE PRISM COVER TEST

The deviation of the two eyes may be measured with the prism cover test. The alternate prism cover test gives the maximum total deviation. One holds prisms in front of one or both eyes (single prisms, prism bars, or rotary prisms) and covers the eyes alternately. If one of the eyes moves out to fixate, the examiner should increase base-out prisms until no refixation movement is noted. If it moves in to fixate, overcorrection is occurring, and the prism strength should be decreased.

Measurements are made with fixation at 6 meters and at 33 centimeters to find the ratio between accommodation and convergence according to the heterophoria method. If there are reasons to suspect incomitance, then the prism cover test may be done at various positions of gaze.

To determine deviation without dissociation, one must do a simultaneous prism cover test. The fixing eye is covered at the same time that an appropriate prism is placed in front of the nonfixing eye. If there is no refixation movement, the deviation equals that of the prism used.

Angle measurements with prisms are associated with a number of errors. Determination of refixation movement is often difficult. Especially with large numbers of prisms, the eye overshoots, resulting in a total movement like that occurring if no prisms are in place. One then sees a movement of redress, the so-called "fixation oscillation."

Holding a prism at an angle changes its values. Nonetheless, the prism cover test gives reliable results. One must always remember, however, that the angle of deviation is not constant but is variable. Furthermore, it is not always necessary to know the exact angle of squint, since surgical intervention cannot be graded that precisely.

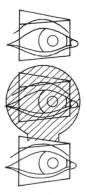
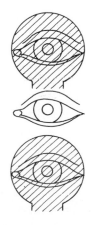

Fig. 34–Alternate prism cover test. Prisms are increased with alternate covers until no further movement is seen.

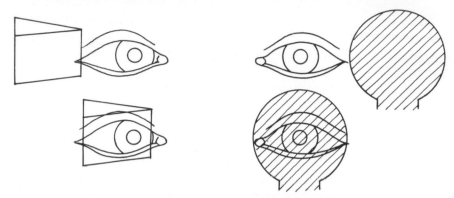

Fig. 35–Simultaneous prism cover test. Simultaneously while covering the fixing eye, one places prisms in front of the nonfixing eye and observes for any refixation movements.

INVESTIGATION OF BINOCULAR VISION

Examination of binocular vision requires knowledge of test results with normal binocular vision and of the alterations with strabismus. Primarily, the question is whether one is dealing with a normal or an abnormal retinal correspondence, whether or not suppression exists, and to what degree. For these examinations, one is dependent upon the subjective answers of the patient.

EXAMINATION WITH BAGOLINI STRIATED GLASSES

Bagolini glasses are plano glasses with finely etched lines. Things are not blurred by the glasses; vision remains unchanged. A point light source, however, is seen as having a fine line radiating from its center. The natural conditions of vision are therefore not altered, and fusion is not interrupted.

Bagolini glasses are placed in front of each eye of the patient so that the lines intersect at a right angle. For example, in front of the right eye, the lines are at 45 degrees, and those in front of the left are at 135 degrees. The patient is then asked to fixate on the light and indicate how the lines of light relate to each other. Various answers can be obtained from this test.

1. The two lines cross at the light, forming an X. Two possibilities exist:
   a. the eyes are parallel, with normal retinal correspondence.
   b. strabismus is present, with harmonious anomalous retinal correspondence. With large-angle deviations, this diagnosis is obvious. If there

is a question of a very small angle of deviation, or of the eyes being parallel, the monocular cover test will make the diagnosis.

2. The patient sees only one line of light, for example, that belonging to the right eye. The left eye is suppressed.

3. Two stripes of light are seen, but one is interrupted near the light source. This indicates a circumscribed zone of suppression or scotoma.
   a. with manifest strabismus, a zero point scotoma with harmonious retinal correspondence.
   b. with the eyes parallel, a central scotoma on the weaker eye, for example, with anisometropia.

4. Two stripes of light are seen, of which only one crosses the light while the other is displaced. This displacement corresponds to the subjective angle of deviation. By turning the Bagolini lens so that the displaced light stripe appears vertically or horizontally, one can then read the vertical or horizontal subjective angle of deviation on the Maddox scale. Two possibilities exist:
   a. Manifest strabismus with normal retinal correspondence: the subjective angle corresponds to the objective angle.
   b. Strabismus with unharmonious anomalous retinal correspondence.

The primary advantage of the Bagolini test is that it is done under normal viewing conditions. This test shows that anomalous retinal correspondence is almost always of the harmonious type, with the exception of cases that have recently undergone a change in the angle of deviation, for example, after surgery.

If one sets the stripes nearly horizontally—for example, the right at 5 degrees and the left at 175 degrees—one can achieve a stereo effect and test stereopsis. The two inferior streaks are fused into a single beam, which comes forward. The superior two divergent beams are fused for a short distance and seen as receding.

We have found that combination of the Bagolini striate glasses test with prisms is useful. For example, if there is a subjective decentration of the lines, these can be recentered with prisms so that they cross at the centered light. The number of prisms employed is useful in determining the surgery to be done.

We have found fusion exercises using striate glasses to be useful in intermittent esotropia or exotropia. Suppression is more easily overcome. The subjective deviation is more easily recognized and may be corrected more readily when one is viewing stripes of light rather than simply a fixation light.

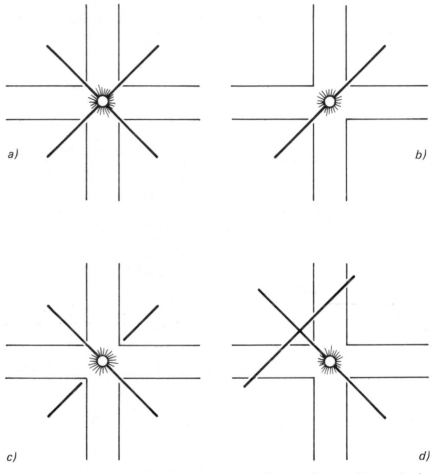

Fig. 36–Bagolini striate lenses. *a*) Light stripes crossing at light: parallel eyes with normal retinal correspondence or strabismus with harmonious anomalous retinal correspondence without a suppression zone. *b*) Suppression of one eye. *c*) Suppression of a stripe of light near the fixation light: central scotoma with straight eyes or a fixation point scotoma with strabismus with harmonious anomalous retinal correspondence. *d*) Shift of a light stripe: strabismus with normal or unharmonious anomalous retinal correspondence.

OPHTHALMOSCOPIC CORRESPONDENCE
TESTING (Method of Cüppers[35])

Ophthalmoscopic testing for retinal correspondence is the most instructive testing method for diagnosis of anomalous retinal correspondence and simultaneously the best way to familiarize oneself with this sensory phenomenon.

The patient fixates, for example, on a light on the Maddox scale with the dominant eye. At the same time, the investigator views the fundus of the other eye through a direct ophthalmoscope, projecting a target whose subjective position in relation to the fixation light must be indicated by the patient. There are two ways of carrying out this test: ophthalmoscopic bifoveal testing and ophthalmoscopic determination of the localization center of anomalous correspondence.

Ophthalmoscopic Bifoveal Testing to Measure Angle of Anomaly

The patient fixates on the light of the tangent scale. The examiner projects the star of the Visuscope onto the fovea of the other eye. The patient must now indicate if the star is seen on the fixation light or next to it.

If the star covers the fixation light, normal retinal correspondence is present. If the star is not seen in the same direction as the fixation light, then the two foveae have a different direction sense, and anomalous retinal correspondence is present. The number on the Maddox scale on which the star is seen gives the angle of anomaly. One must first project the star and then ask where it is seen. Otherwise, the patient will attempt to look at the star, thereby shifting fixation.

Ophthalmoscopic Determination of the Localization Center of Anomalous Correspondence

One shifts the Visuscope star in the fundus until it is seen to be in the same direction as the fixation light. This point represents the localization center of the anomalous retinal correspondence or the anomaly center. This point is sometimes called pseudomacula, a term best avoided because it may be confused with eccentric fixation.

Determination of the localization center is more difficult than determination of the angle of anomaly, since the localization center is usually suppressed more strongly than the fovea. Here one finds zero point scotoma. Often, the patient will indicate that the star disappears as soon as it gets near the fixation light. In a sense, one can do perimetry directly on the fundus in this way to get information regarding scotoma size.

The star should be displaced in the fundus upward and to the side, out of the scotoma. The patient is asked when the star is directly below the light. The correspondence center is directly above this in the fundus. The answers have to make sense in terms of distance and direction indicated.

With an angle deviation of 15 degrees, one frequently finds that the scotoma encroaches upon the disc. (See blind-spot mechanism according to Swan.)

The advantages of this method are its direct visibility, objectivity, and possibility of rechecking answers. Bifoveal testing in this way is the examination method of choice with small-angle deviations and with eccentric fixation. The drawbacks are that the patient must be a good observer in order

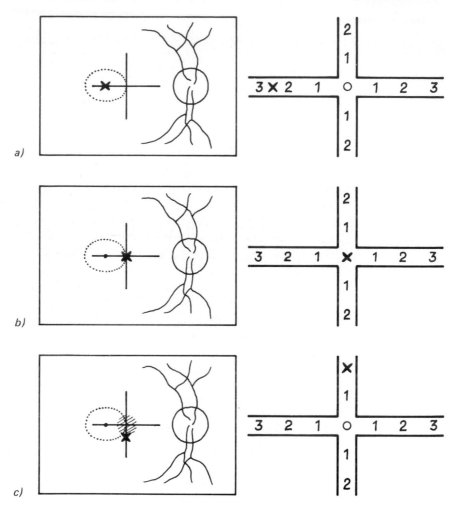

Fig. 37–Ophthalmoscopic correspondence testing: a Visuscope star is projected into the right eye and the left eye fixates on a light: *a*) The star projected onto the fovea is seen to the left of straight ahead: esotropia, anomalous retinal correspondence, with an angle of anomaly of 2 1/2 degrees. *b*) The star is seen binocularly as straight ahead in the localization center of anomalous retinal correspondence and lies in the same direction as the fixation light. *c*) With a fixation point scotoma one moves the star out of the scotoma until it is seen as directly over the light. X indicates fixation. ● indicates center of correspondence

to give exact answers. For this reason, the method is almost impossible to carry out with children. It is also not useful for patients with alternate suppression.

With large-scale deviations, the investigation is carried out by placing a mirror in front of the fixing eye at a 45-degree angle. The patient then fixates on the light on the Maddox cross via this mirror. With smaller angle deviations, a prism base can be placed in front of the fixing eye. In this way, the examiner's head does not obstruct fixation.

We ourselves use a periscope like a double-mirror viewer (Fig. 38). We routinely examine in this way on the Maddox scale at five meters' distance, especially with microstrabismus. The advantage of this method is that the Maddox scale does not appear to be reversed right to left, and, therefore, one does not have to rethink the responses concerning the center of location. If the Visuscope star is suppressed because of its small size, one needs a larger target.

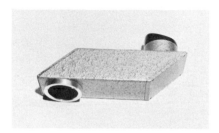

Fig. 38–Double mirror viewer.

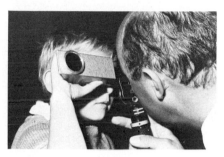

Fig. 39–Correspondence testing ophthalmoscopically with the Visuscope and the double mirror viewer.

EXAMINATION WITH THE WORTH FOUR DOT LIGHT TEST[140]

The patient wears red/green glasses and looks at four lights arranged in a cross with the two horizontal lights being green, the top light red, and the bottom light white.

With normal binocular vision the patient sees four lights, one red above, two green on each side, and a pale red underneath. Occasionally, with harmonious anomalous retinal correspondence, four lights are also seen. This is especially true with microstrabismus. In the latter, the size of the cross made by the lights and the distance of the lights from each other are important in that they relate to the size of the suppression scotoma. For example, Worth lights, whose total size is 17.5 centimeters, form an angle of two degrees when viewed at five meters' distance. If viewed from one meter's distance, this angle is nine degrees. This means that the scotoma is at least the size of this object.

If the patient sees either two red or three green lights, one eye is suppressed.

The angle of convergence often increases with red/green glasses because Worth lights are strongly dissociating and deviate from the normal conditions of viewing. Therefore, it is not uncommon to find anomalous retinal correspondence of unharmonious type.

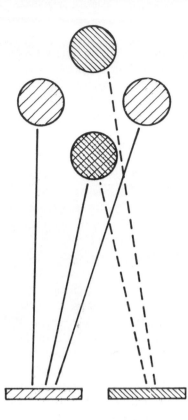

Fig. 40–Worth four-dot test: the two horizontal lights are green; the top light is red, the lower light is white. Red is in front of the right eye, green in front of the left.

EXAMINATION WITH HERING AFTERIMAGES

Examination of afterimages serves to differentiate between normal and anomalous retinal correspondence. The patient fixates on a vertically oriented light stripe with his right eye; his left eye is occluded. Subsequently, a horizontal light stripe is fixated by his left eye, with the right eye occluded. This produces horizontal or vertical afterimages in the respective eyes. The patient is then asked to close both eyes and subsequently to look at a blank background, preferably with strong flickering illumination. The patient sees the afterimages of the two light sources. At first, the afterimages appear as bright lines (positive afterimages), later on as dark lines (negative afterimages). If the two afterimages are seen as a cross, normal retinal correspondence exists. With anomalous retinal correspondence, the two lines are displaced relative to each other, for example, as a reclining T. This displacement occurs because with anomalous retinal correspondence, the two foveae do not have the same visual direction.

The light source for the afterimages can be a special tube light or a flash of light with the appropriate shields. Afterimages can also be introduced on the

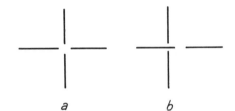

Fig. 41–Hering's afterimages.

a) Cross with normal retinal correspondence; and

b) Displacement with anomalous retinal correspondence.

synoptophore. The size of the afterimages is important. Large afterimages can cover up small angles of anomaly. Synoptophore afterimages of 10 degrees (Clemment & Clark) and 14 degrees (Oculus) are commercially available.

EXAMINATION WITH A DARK RED GLASS OR THE MADDOX ROD

While the patient fixates on a point light source, one places a dark red glass or Maddox rod in front of one eye. The Maddox rod consists of a number of parallel rods or cylinders. These will change a point light source to a streak that is perpendicular to the direction of the rods in the cylinder. Through the dark red glass or the Maddox rod, the fixation light can be seen, but not its surroundings. Fusion is therefore totally suspended. If the red light is seen on the white fixation light, or in the case of the Maddox rod, if the red streak of light crosses the white light subjectively, there is no deviation. This is the case with straight eyes, with normal retinal correspondence, or with manifest strabismus if harmonious anomalous retinal correspondence exists.

With esophoria, uncrossed diplopia is noted. This means that with a red glass in front of the left eye, the red light is seen to the left of the white fixation light. One can also speak of same-sided or homonymous diplopia.

With exophoria, crossed or heteronomous diplopia is seen. For example, while the patient is fixing on a white light with a red glass in front of the left eye, the dark red light appears to the right of the white fixation light.

Right hypophoria (or left hyperphoria) is present if with the red glass in front of the right eye, the red light is seen above the white. If the red light is seen below the white, there is right hyperphoria (left hypophoria).

This examination can be done using two types of fixation. If the eye without the red filter is fixing, then the red light falls on a nonfoveal retinal area in the other eye. The red light is then localized in space by the corresponding retinal area of the free (nonfiltered) eye. For example, with esotropia of seven degrees with the free (nonfiltered) right eye fixing, the red light falls on an eccentric retinal area seven degrees nasal in the (red filtered) left eye. The corresponding temporal retinal area of the free right eye then localizes the red light in space seven degrees to the left of the fixation light.

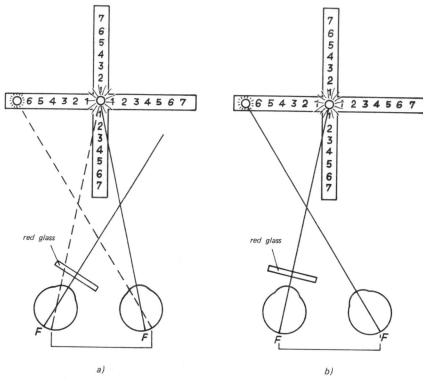

Fig. 42–Examination with the red glass in esotropia: homonymous or uncrossed diplopia: *a*) The right eye fixes on the white light. In the left eye, the red light falls on a nasal retinal area. This corresponds with a temporal retinal area in the right eye, which then localizes the red light to the left. *b*) The left eye has a red glass in front of it and fixates on the light. The fovea of the left eye corresponding with the fovea of the right eye localizes the light to the left at the degree of deviation. *c*) The Lang Stereo test based on the principle of panography.

One can have the patient demonstrate this deviation on a tangent scale. The amount of prism needed to do this gives the degree of deviation. This type of measurement is called "recentration."

The deviation can be measured by placing a prism in front of the red filter, shifting the red light so that it is superimposed on top of the white. Then the patient will usually change fixation.

When the light is fixed, with the eye having the red glass in front of it, the fovea of the free eye localizes the red light in space. For example, if one is dealing with esotropia of seven degrees and finds the red glass in front of the left fixing eye, then the right eye is in a convergent position of seven degrees. With its fovea, it localizes the red light seven degrees to the left of the fixation light. This is called the "reading-off" method.

With the recentration method, the red light is sometimes not seen because it may fall into a suppresion area on the fundus. With vertical prisms, it can be shifted out of this suppression region and recognized.

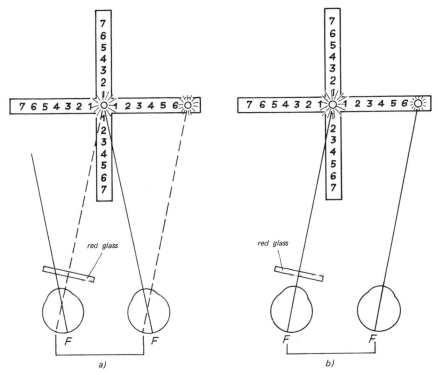

Fig. 43–Examination with the red glass with exotropia: heteronymous or crossed localization: *a)* The right eye fixates the light. In the left eye the red light falls onto a temporal retinal area which corresponds with the nasal retinal area of the right eye which localizes the red light to the right. *b)* The left eye which has a red glass in front of it fixates the light. The fovea of the right eye localizes the light corresponding to the angle of deviation to right.

With the recentration method, one needs not a tangent scale but prisms. For the reading-off method, a tangent scale is useful. One can ask the patient to point at the red light with a pointer. With small angles, one may measure at a distance of five meters (with larger angles, at one meter) where the small numbers of the tangent scale are used. Tangent scales also exist for use at other distances. During the examination, attention is paid to the position of the eyes. Fixation can change spontaneously. Usually, fixation occurs first with the free eye, but in an effort to read off the deviation, it shifts to the eye behind the red glass. In muscle paresis, fixation is almost always with the red glass eye.

Localization of the red light is always opposite to the eye position. With esotropia, the axis of the eyes is crossed, and localization is uncrossed. With exotropia, the axes of the eyes are not crossed, the images are crossed. With incyclophoria, the eye is intorted, and the Maddox rod line is tilted out. With excyclophoria, the eye is rotated out, the Maddox rod line in. Torsion is best diagnosed by placing a white Maddox rod lens in front of the right eye vertically and a red Maddox rod in front of the left eye vertically. With a vertical deviation, one then sees two lines and determines whether or not they are parallel. As a rule, one should ophthalmologically check the position of the fovea in relationship to the disc.

EXAMINATION WITH A MADDOX WING

The Maddox wing is used for examination at near gaze. The instrument is 32 centimeters long and is held by a handle. With both eyes open, one looks at a plate on which a vertical and a horizontal row of numbers and a white arrow have been printed. A red arrow is mounted so that it is moveable. The visual impressions of the two eyes are dissociated by means of a central divider. The right eye sees the horizontal row of numbers, while the left eye sees the arrow. The position of the white arrow in relation to the numbers gives the horizontal deviation in prism diopters. Vertical deviation is recognized by the position of the horizontal red arrow in relation to a vertical row of numbers. Cyclophoria is recognized in the shift of the horizontal arrow in relationship to a horizontal line. The degree of torsion can be read off on a scale.

COORDIMETRY HESS SCREEN TESTING

Vertical and horizontal lines are located at five-degree intervals on a screen with a fixation point in the center. Eight further fixation points at an interval of 15 degrees form an inner quadrant. An outer quadrant is marked by points at 30-degree intervals. The patient puts his chin on the chin rest 50 centimeters from the screen and wears red/green glasses. He is asked to fixate on the central red point and the points of the inner quadrant one after the other while localizing these using a green pointer. Through the red/green glasses, he sees the red points with the right eye and localizes the green points with the left eye.

In the original version, the red marks were on a dark cloth, and the patient used a dark pointer with a green mark on its tip to localize the red mark. The more modern versions use red and green projection lights. This method is excellent for testing eye muscle paresis. Over and underaction of muscles is graphically illustrated.

The Hess screen was modified over time so that with the Lees screen, instead of the color dissociation, a mirror is used with two Hess screens at right angles to each other. With the Lancaster modification, the patient sits at a distance of one meter from the screen. Here, the measurement used is prism diopters; angle degrees are used with the Hess screen. For this reason, the Lancaster screen has straight lines, while the Hess screen's lines are concave toward the center. The individual lines are usually five centimeters from each other, thereby measuring five prism diopters.

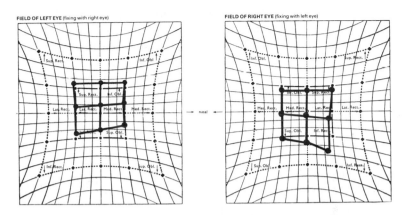

Fig. 44–Example of Hess screen testing. Paresis of the left superior oblique with overaction of the right inferior rectus. Shown are the Lancaster screen, the Foster, the Lees, and the Hess-Weiss. Normal retinal correspondence is prerequisite to getting correct responses to these tests.

BINOCULAR FIELD OF FIXATION TESTING FOR DIPLOPIA

The evaluation of the symptoms of subjective diplopia is of particular importance for insurance compensation purposes. Here the size of the area of diplopia is of special interest. The Hess screen, like all other dissociated forms of examination, is not suited for this purpose. More useful is binocular examination using a bowl perimeter. The chin rest is placed in the center, and the patient is asked to fixate on the moving light target with both eyes. In this way, the areas of single and double vision are readily marked, and the course of healing can be documented for comparison purposes. One can begin the examination from the area of diplopia or from the area of fusion. The comparison of the two gives information about the functional range.

Normally, the binocular visual fields extend 50 degrees across, 40 degrees superiorly, and 60 degrees inferiorly. The useful visual field for daily life is restricted to about 15 to 20 degrees.

EXAMINATION ON THE SYNOPTOPHORE (MAJOR AMBLYOSCOPE)

The synoptophore consists of two tubes at an angle to each other, thus placing a picture in front of each eye. The tubes are moveable so that any angle of deviation can be obtained. Introduction of seven-diopter convex lenses into the oculars relaxes accommodation, and the picture which is at 14.3 centimeters is seen as if were at infinity.

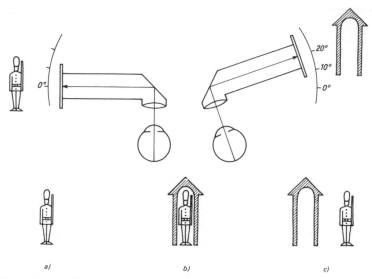

a)   b)   c)

Fig. 45–Examination of the patient with convergence strabismus on the Synoptophore. The arms of the Synoptophore are adjusted for an objective angle of 20 degrees. *a*) The patient suppresses the picture of the right eye. *b*) Simultaneous vision occurs at the objective angle. *c*) The guard house is seen to the left of the soldier.

The subjective angle does not correspond with the objective angle. Anomalous retinal correspondence exists. The fovea of the right eye in binocular vision has the visual direction of left of straight ahead.

The patient is seated at the synoptophore, and the chin and forehead rest are so adjusted that the eyes are at the level of the oculars, about 1.5 centimeters from them. The examiner should be able to see the patient's corneal reflex. The arms of the synoptophore are set for the interpupillary distance.

MEASUREMENT OF THE OBJECTIVE ANGLE OF DEVIATION

If central fixation is present, one places one synoptophore arm at zero and the other at the presumed angle of deviation. Small pictures are used to assure central fixation. As with the unilateral alternating cover test or the simultaneous or alternating prism cover test, two methods of investigation are possible.

In the first, both pictures are illuminated. The patient is asked to fixate on the center of one picture. Then this picture is shut off, and the examiner observes whether the other eye makes a fixation movement. If this is the case, the process is repeated and the synoptophore arms are shifted until no fixation movement is visible. Between each phase of the examination, both pictures are illuminated so that binocular vision is possible. This method is equivalent to the monocular cover test or the simultaneous prism cover test.

In the second variation, both pictures are shown alternately, and the synoptophore arms are adjusted until no refixation movement develops. This method is equivalent to the alternate cover test and the alternate prism cover test, since no binocular vision is possible. With this method, the angle of deviation is often greater. Horizontal deviations are compensated for by moving the synoptophore arms, vertical deviations by elevating or depressing the synoptophore pictures.

When one eye is deeply amblyopic without the capacity for fixation, one can determine an objective angle of deviation by shifting the synoptophore arm in front of the amblyopic eye until the corneal reflex is centered in the pupil.

THE SUBJECTIVE EXAMINATION

In testing simultaneous pictures, the pair of pictures used is totally different—for example, a soldier and a guard house. The patient should shift the Synoptophore arm until the soldier is seen to be in the guard house. If this subjective angle coincides with the measured objective angle, then normal retinal correspondence exists. If these angles do not correspond, then anomalous retinal correspondence is present. With harmonious anomalous retinal correspondence, the subjective angle is zero degrees.

With unharmonious retinal correspondence, the subjective angle is usually between zero degrees and the objective angle. Suppression is common at the subjective angle, or the patient may see the images alternately. The area of suppression is equivalent to the zero point scotoma. Sometimes the deviating eye is totally suppressed.

Fusion pictures consist of a pair of similar images, each of which has a different control. For example, in one picture a boy holds flowers in his right hand, but in the other picture he has a watering can in the left hand. Fusion exists when the patient sees only one boy but with both the flowers and the watering can. Starting at the angle of fusion, the divergence and convergence can be measured for the fusional range.

Finally, stereoscopic pictures can be used to test stereopsis. Examination at the synoptophore can be combined with testing of entoptic phenomena—for example, Haidinger brushes or afterimages.

In order to interpret synoptophore findings, one must keep in mind that the objective angle in esotropia is usually greater at the synoptophore than in free space. Consequently, one detects unharmonious anomalous retinal correspondence more often. For example, if at the synoptophore the objective angle is +30 degrees and the subjective angle +10 degrees, one can assume that in free space an angle of +20 degrees with a subjective angle of 0 degrees is present.

The strabismic angle can vary at the synoptophore. Frequently, the convergence angle increases during objective measurement (alternating presentation) and decreases during subjective measurement (simultaneous presentation). In this way, the measured angle of anomaly is too large. With microtropia, we therefore always first determine the subjective angle of deviation and only thereafter the objective. One should constantly monitor the eye position.

EXAMINATION FOR STEREOPSIS

Stereopsis or depth perception is the highest degree of binocular vision. A rough form of depth sensation is possible monocularly through perspective, shadows, spatial relationships of various objects to each other, and parallax. Useful binocular stereopsis is also present in manifest deviations with anomalous retinal correspondence. In this case, however, the degree of depth perception usually is very low. Stereoscopy exists when one presents separate haploscopic images to each eye with different horizontal disparities. Test methods with natural viewing such as the three rod test, Hering's experiment, the Frisby test, and the pointing test can be employed for stereopsis.

THE TWO PENCIL TEST [95]

The test involving touching two pencils quickly orients one about practical depth perception. The patient holds a pencil with the blunt end down and attempts to touch a second pencil with it that the examiner is holding blunt end up at eye level. First this is attempted with both eyes open, then with one eye closed. In this way, the ability to hit a target is tested under monocular and binocular conditions. It is amazing how much even an amblyopic eye helps with binocular vision. The peripheral retinal areas play a large role here. A pencil 17 cm long at a distance of 33 cm has a height of 27 arc degrees. A foveal scotoma in this situation does not act as negatively as it does with other types of stereo testing. The positional disparity can be recognized even with the periphery of the weaker eye and compensated for. With a tubular visual field, the opposite is true. There are therefore a whole series of circumstances in which the touching test is useful:

— with harmonious anomalous retinal correspondence, the test is done better binocularly than monocularly.
— in late-onset normosensorial strabismus and all types of strabismus in which binocularity has been lost, the binocular touch test is poor.
— with eye muscle palsies, one can use the touch test to determine in which direction of gaze binocular vision is present, where suppression or double vision occurs, and why a head turn exists.
— when monocularity has been present since birth, the touch test is usually very good; with acquired monocularity, however, it is bad.

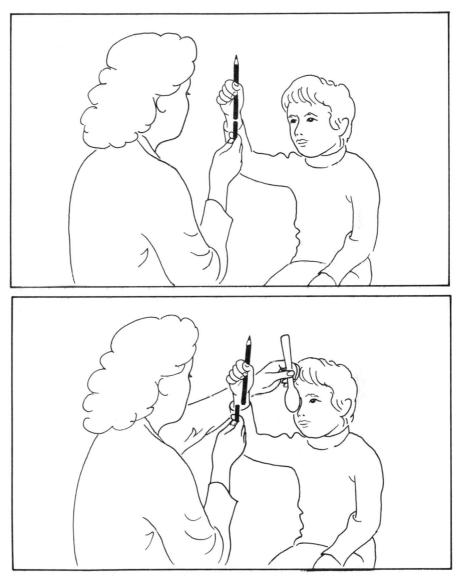

Fig. 46–Pointing test. The patient attempts to touch a pencil, first with both eyes open, then with one eye covered.

— with unilateral cataracts, even with vision as low as 0.1 diopters and less, the ability to touch with both eyes open is much better than it is covering the weaker eye. This may determine whether a cataract operation is indicated.

The pencil touch test is also useful for visual training—for example, to improve the visual field or convergence postoperatively. The stereoscopic requirements act more forcibly on motor fusional innervation than does simple simultaneous viewing or fusional stimulation.

THE PULFRICH PHENOMENON

A neutral-density filter is placed in front of one eye while the subject views a moving pendulum binocularly. There is a sensation of depth: The pendulum appears to be moving in a circle. This is induced by decreased illumination in one eye.

EXAMINATION WITH STEREOSCOPIC PICTURES

Separate pictures are presented to each eye. Because they are slightly disparate they can be fused, thereby eliciting stereopsis. This can be done with the Synoptophore, with the stereoscope, with polarized glasses (Vectograph), or with the use of red/green glasses. One can measure the threshold of stereoscopic vision by determining the degree of disparity being viewed.

A very popular test based upon polarized lighting is the Titmus test. With polarized glasses, a fly appears three-dimensionally; the wing tips have a disparity of 3800 seconds of arc. A series of circles with decreasing displacements allows testing of depth perception up to 40 seconds of arc. Besides those stereo tests that have contours, the stereo test based on a system of random dots as per Julesz has recently become popular. These have the advantages that they allow no monocular clues, and that their forms can be seen only with intact binocularity.

The TNO test is based on a red/green differentiation. Disparity ranges from 1980 down to 15 angle seconds. The random-dot test is based on Vectography and ranges from 600 to 20 seconds of arc. At a distance of 40 cm, the random "E" test has a disparity of 630 seconds of arc. On increasing the distance, this disparity becomes smaller.

With all these tests, one has to wear either red/green or polarized glasses. This is not true with the following test.

The Frisby test consists of three plates which are 6 mm, 3 mm, and 1 mm thick, respectively. A random-dot pattern is printed on one side and a small circular segment on the back side. The angle of disparity is 495, 250, and 85 seconds of arc, respectively.

We have developed a new test, the Lang stereo test, which is particularly useful in testing small children.[94] The separation of the pictures is based on the grid of cylinders of W.R. Hess. Three pictures are presented: a cat with a disparity of 1200 seconds of arc, a star with 600 seconds of arc disparity, and a car with 550 seconds of arc disparity. Examination is very quick. Small children, sometimes even infants, see the figures. This can be determined by observing their eye movements.

There is not only a quantitative but also a qualitative difference between contour stereograms and random-dot stereograms. Patients with amblyopia ex anisometropia recognize the random-dot stereograms, whereas microtropes do not recognize them as well but will recognize contour.

THE PRISM BALANCE TEST OF GRAEFE

The Graefe test is performed in two steps. A six-diopter base-up prism is placed in front of one eye to evoke vertical diplopia. If these double images are not directly one above the other (they are usually also shifted horizontally), additional horizontal prisms are added until the images are one above the other. This provides the degree of heterophoria. For vertical heterophoria, one can place a 10-diopter base-in prism in front of one eye. This shifts the images horizontally. If these also appear displaced vertically, a vertical deviation is present, which can be measured using appropriate prisms.

The Phoroptor with built-in dissociating prisms and a rotary prism is a useful instrument for measurement at both distance and near gaze.

HAPLOSCOPIC EXAMINATION WITH PROJECTORS

There are a number of test-chart projectors that can be used simultaneously with vectographs or the red/glass anaglyph method to test binocular vision (A.O. Mollere, and so forth).

An instrument specifically designed for examining binocular vision is the phase-difference haploscope of Aulhorn. With this, separate images are presented to both eyes at a rate of 50 times per second.

For years, we have used a Vivid stereo projector (Chicago), which was used to view stereo photographs more than 50 years ago. We use copies of synoptophore plates, Amsler grids, and slides of the Lang stereo test. For small children, it is particularly useful to present these at a distance of several meters.

The Pola test of Zeiss contains binocularly different polarized images that are retroilluminated. The Vectograph consists of four polarized test pictures viewed through polarized glasses. With the cross test, one eye sees two vertical lines, the other two horizontal lines that binocularly are seen as a cross with a small central free zone. With heterophoria, this cross is displaced. With suppression, only one of the cross lines is seen. The cyclophoria test shows torsion through the oblique position of one of the cross lines. The aniseikonia test consists of a binocularly seen central ring with two monocularly seen half-quadrants on either side. With aniseikonia, these appear to be different sizes. With the stereo test, the sensation of depth is achieved through two displaced triangles. Proponents of the polarized light test claim that the findings can be directly translated into prism corrections in the glasses. There is difference of opinion on this point.[12,57]

THE FOUR-DIOPTER BASE-OUT PRISM
TEST[73]

A four-diopter base-out prism is placed in front of one eye. The eye behind the prism must make an adducting movement of four diopters to maintain fixation. The examiner observes the other eye. When it is suppressed, it makes an abducting movement of four diopters but then stays in that position. When fusion is present, this abduction movement is corrected through a slow convergence movement. The same procedure is then repeated with the other eye. With microstrabismus or amblyopia ex anisometropia, frequently this fusional movement does not take place or takes place very slowly. One therefore cannot differentiate between these two conditions by use of the four-diopter base-out prism test. It is useful in all cases to hold up the prism's base in.

3

TYPES OF STRABISMUS AND DISTURBANCES IN MOTILITY

Prerequisite for correct diagnosis is a thorough knowledge of the various disturbances of ocular motility and testing techniques. Division of strabismus into paralytic and concomitant types is useful, as is the categorizing into esotropia, exotropia, and vertical deviations. Manifest strabismus can be differentiated from latent strabismus (heterophoria). Strabismus may be unilateral or alternating, with or without amblyopia. It may be constant or intermittent. If it is intermittent, it can be greater either at near gaze or at distance and may have a very specific rhythmic pattern.

Further subdivisions of strabismus can be made depending on the size of the angle (see later), the type of sensory disturbances (anomalous correspondence, amblyopia), and the refraction (high hyperopia, emmetropia, anisometropia, myopia). Even so-called concomitant strabismus can show a degree of incomitance, for example with variable horizontal angles, according to the vertical gaze ("A" and "V" patterns), or incomitance of the vertical deviation according to the direction of horizontal gaze. The term "anisotropia" means that the angle of deviation varies depending on which eye fixes. With all these variations, one should still attempt to differentiate each case of strabismus by other criteria.

There are various typical strabismus syndrome types that one should know. Quite characteristic is the combination of the congenital squint syndrome, microstrabismus, full accommodative strabismus, and the normo sensorial late onset strabismus. Frequently, in individual cases various factors interplay with each other so that combinations of different types are present.

Therefore, all classifications are somewhat subjective. To deal with the complexity of the field, a systematic subdivision into types of strabismus is necessary while retaining as broad an overview as possible.

HETEROPHORIA

Heterophoria is defined as a latent deviation compensated for by fusion. With interruption of fusion, the eyes deviate into their fusion-free position of rest. If this position of rest is convergent, one has esophoria; if divergent, exophoria. Vertical positions of rest elicit hyper- or hypophoria. Cyclophoria is rotation around the sagittal axis.

Orthophoria is present when the eyes remain in a parallel position, even with suspension of fusion. This is rare and usually occurs only with short interruptions of fusion, as with the cover test. If fusion is interrupted for longer periods of time, for example with occlusion therapy, heterophorias are the rule and orthophoria is the exception. Anatomic, optical, and innervational factors determine the fusion-free position of rest.

The anatomic content of the orbits varies structurally and includes muscles, fascia, and fat. Despite such anatomic variability, the eyes are generally parallel.

Optical causes of heterophoria include any factors leading to blurred vision. This includes opacities of the optical media, severe refractive errors including severe astigmatism and aphakia, and an unclear image. Aniseikonia, a difference in image size, also leads to a weakness of fusion.

Owing to an excessive need for accommodation, hyperopic refractive errors can lead to esophoria. The lack of accommodation with myopia may lead to exophoria.

Among innervational factors, there is a differentiation between negative and positive factors. Those that disrupt the parallel position are negative. Those that aid in maintaining parallelism are positive.

Convergence tone is a major negative factor in esotropia. Chronic convergence is especially prominent in small children and can be increased by emotions such as anger or embarrassment. In exotropia, convergence is useful and a positive factor.

The most important factor that compensates for heterophoria is fusion. This may be present in varying degrees. It is amazing how large a heterophoric deviation can be compensated for, without symptoms, by fusion so long as the physiologic and psychic condition of the patient is healthy. Generalized debility or illness, fatigue, decreased attention span, or a decline in the optical quality of vision all lead to a decrease in fusional capacity. Typical of this type of fusional disturbance are those occurring after head trauma with cerebral contusion and those associated with alcoholic intoxication. These can lead to diplopia.

Heterophoria-induced complaints are very difficult to evaluate. Generally, one speaks of asthenopic symptoms, which may include headaches, fatigue, burning, photophobia, and blurred vision. Such complaints can also be caused by other factors including conjunctivitis, uncorrected refractive error, and early presbyopia.

Patients with cervical migraine especially complain about periorbital headaches combined with difficulty in reading. This leads to an intensive and prolonged search for refractive errors or heterophorias. In order not to overlook a cervical syndrome, one should make it a rule to ask about occipital headaches, dizziness, and pain radiating into the arms. The occipital headaches are typically described by the patient as radiating from the back of the head forward. In his description, the patient will make a motion with his hands, as if taking off a helmet. A certain sign that complaints are heterophoria-induced is that symptoms are alleviated by eye closure. One has to ask about this in the history.

Individual disposition to headaches is also important. There are patients in whom the smallest problem leads to severe headaches, while others don't even know what headaches are. Such patients do not get headaches, even after a typical migraine flicker scotoma.

Psychic disposition plays a large role in heterophoria. In this sense, it is difficult to differentiate how much the patient has been psychologically changed by his years of complaints, or if the psychologic disturbance is primary to the complaints and the heterophoria is only a minor component.

In the evaluation of heterophoric patients, the history, general physical condition, and eye findings must all be considered.

Examination for heterophoria should determine the degree of disease and the effect of compensatory mechanisms. Such an examination can be very time-consuming and may require several sittings, potentially at different times of the day.

The simplest and most informative examination is the cover test. The alternate cover test shows the type and degree of deviation and the form of compensation. The deviation can be measured at distance and near gaze with prisms. The uncover test reveals how the patient compensates for this latent deviation. A rapid refusion movement during the uncover test indicates good fusion, whereas a very slow or prolonged refixation movement indicates a disturbance in either the sensory or the motor component of the fusion mechanism.

Further measurement of heterophoria can be done with dark red glasses or the Maddox's rod at a distance using a tangent scale. The Maddox wing is very useful for near measurements. Cyclophorias can be measured in space using a trial frame with different-colored Maddox rods in front of each eye.

With these techniques, the deviation of the eyes can be quantitated. Recentration can be measured by placing prisms in front of the eyes as therapy. The Vectographic projection test and the Graefe test are common ways of measuring recentration. Equally easy is the testing of heterophorias on the synoptophore. Not only the range of fusion but also rotation can be readily measured. In free space, the fusional range can be measured with prisms (prism bars, rotary prisms).

Fusional range is measured starting at the null point. More convergent or divergent prisms are added by moving the synoptophore arm until double vision occurs. With the eyes converging, a point is reached at which the image becomes smaller. Here the convergence movement is inducing accommodation even though the distance of the fixation object remains unchanged. Thus, the fusional amplitude has two components: convergence without accommodation and convergence with accommodation. Graphically, this point is where the fusion line suddenly rises. The range of fusion with accommodation lies between the blur point and the point where fusion breaks into diplopia.

In addition to measuring the fusional amplitudes starting at zero to the breaking point, one should also measure away from the region of diplopia back to that point where it disappears (refusion or recovery point). This point tells us as much about fusional capacity as do fusional amplitudes. All these values can be illustrated graphically according to the method of Donders.

Normal values for fusional amplitudes vary according to direction. They range 10 to 20 degrees for convergence, 4 to 6 degrees for divergence, and 1 to 2 degrees for vertical fusion. Cyclophorias up to 15 degrees can be overcome. Motor compensation does not account for the full 15 degrees but only a small fraction thereof. The remainder is compensated for purely sensorially.

It is amazing how large a heterophoric deviation can be compensated for with heterophoria. One can find esophoria and hyperphoria of 10 degrees or more that are compensated. In other words, amplitudes of divergence and vertical vergence of more than 10 degrees have developed. Amplitudes of this extent are rarely seen in these directions in normal eyes. The reason for this is that in casual gaze, there are no instances in which fusion has to be maintained to overcome divergence of a vertical deviation of that degree, and this is therefore not practiced. With greater demands comes an increase in the ability to do this. As a rule, people have the amount of fusional capacity that they need.

If heterophorias cause no symptoms, treatment is unnecessary. If complaints exist, however, it is always a question whether these may be related to the heterophoria or due to other factors. For this reason, one does not recommend comprehensive therapy with only one consultation but starts with symptomatic treatment. First, all refractive errors that may play a role in heterophoria are eliminated. Symptomatic therapy can vary from case to case, including such things as use of bland eyedrops and massaging of the forehead and base of the neck.

An exact refractive correction is recommended. A small "plus" correction for close work or a light tint for photosensitivity may be useful. The need for cycloplegic examination varies from case to case. We take the position that cycloplegic examination should always be carried out in adults before prismatic correction is prescribed.

Prismatic correction in heterophoria is a very controversial subject. A sensible conclusion is often difficult to reach. On one side is the opinion that prisms should never be prescribed. The other is that heterophoria should be corrected prismatically. Universal rules do not apply here, and no single investigative technique can replace the experience and clinical bias of the examiner.

The easiest cases to correct are those in which heterophoria is induced through use of incorrect glasses. Large frames frequently result in a larger distance between optical centers. Use of temporally decentered glasses may lead to esophoria in severe myopes and to exophoria in hyperopes. The optical center and interpupillary distance must always be checked.

Conversely, one can utilize this effect by decentering the glasses in esophoria nasally in myopes and temporally in hyperopes. With exophoria, one should decenter nasally in hyperopes and temporally in myopes. The prismatic effect of decentration is limited and is dependent upon the strength of the glasses. Each centimeter of decentration per diopter of glasses strength produces one prism diopter.

Induced prism by decentration = decentration (in cm) x strength of the lens (in diopters)

A myopic correction of five diopters decentered five millimeters gives a deviation of 2.5 prism diopters. Larger deviations must be corrected by prescribing prisms.

The prescription of prisms has its limits in that prisms shift the images, produce schematic aberrations, and are cosmetically unattractive, expensive, and heavy. On top of this, it is not rare that after prolonged use of corrective prisms, the original complaints return, and the prism correction has to be increased to the point where surgery is required. Prisms should therefore never be prescribed without clear indications and purpose.

Through internal reflection, prisms can induce diplopia. The second image is displaced six times the prism strength and is attenuated by 99.8%. Weak prisms worn bilaterally will create a disturbing binocular triplopia when bright punctate light sources are viewed. This phenomenon is not common knowledge, but it should be recognized and understood. It can be prevented with antireflective treatment of the prisms.

The prism bends the light toward its base. An object seen through the prism appears to be displaced in the direction of the apex. With esodeviation, we prescribe prisms that are base out; with exodeviation, base in (nasal). To minimize the optical distortions and schematic aberrations, it is useful to divide the total number of prisms needed between the two eyes (for example, four diopters base out for each eye). The same is true for vertical prisms. With six diopters of right hypertropia, one prescribes three diopters base down for the right eye and three diopters base up for the left eye. Oblique prisms can be recalculated into their vertical and horizontal components. For example, six diopters on a base of 120 degrees is equivalent to seven diopters at base 90 plus five diopters at base 180. Instead of prescribing four prism diopters at 180 degrees and seven prism diopters at 90 degrees, one can use eight prism diopters at 60 degrees to achieve the same effect (Fig. 47).

In individual cases, exercises with prisms in free space or at the synoptophore may be useful. These exercises increase the fusional amplitudes, improve fusional movements, or minimize suppression. Here, too, a degree of caution is needed, in that such exercises may lead to a worsening of symptoms.

With large heterophorias, surgery may be indicated. There is a great gap in the literature concerning indications for and effect of heterophoria operations. With esophoria, it has been our experience that unilateral recession of the medial rectus muscle gives little result. On the other hand, a recession resection leads to restriction of adduction in esophoria, even with very careful measurements. Nonetheless, with well-motivated patients, such surgery is often very much appreciated. The surgical indication is less troublesome in those cases in which heterophoria has a tendency toward tropia. An example of this is exophoria, which has a tendency to decompensate into intermittent exotropia.

Convergence insufficiency must be classified with heterophoria. It is hallmarked by an inability to converge both eyes normally or to maintain

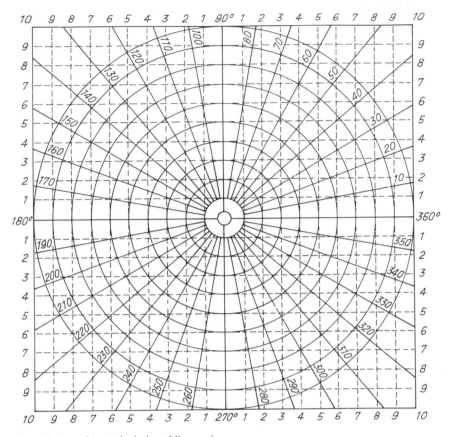

Fig. 47–Schema for recalculating oblique prisms.

convergence over long periods of time. There is an entire spectrum of these types of conditions, ranging from true convergence palsies to posttraumatic convergence insufficiency, to a minimal decrease in covergence with presbyopia, to temporal decentration of "plus" lenses. A large interpupillary distance seems to predispose one to convergence insufficiencies.

The near point of convergence is normally six centimeters. With convergence insufficiency, one eye deviates before this. Subjectively, this deviation may result in diplopia. A very useful method for subjective measurement of convergence is the "near point rule:" The alternate prism cover test at near gaze shows a significantly greater exophoria than at a distance. In Donder's diagram, this is seen as a steep convergence line.

Accommodative deficiency often accompanies convergence insufficiency. One therefore also has to measure the near point of accommodation.

Orthoptic treatment of convergence insufficiency is very successful. Exercises for recognition of physiologic diplopia are carried out with stereograms. The primary convergence exercise is called "push-ups." A small fixation object is repeatedly brought closer and closer to the nose. Convergence exercises utilizing the Bagolini glasses are very useful, since the patient can check convergence on the basis of the crossing streaks of light. Also, practicing the two-pencil touch test has advantages because the use of stereopsis stimulates the convergence impulse.

ESSENTIAL STRABISMUS AND NORMO-SENSORIAL LATE-ONSET STRABISMUS

The term "essential" indicates that there is no known cause. One is dealing neither with congenital nor with accommodative strabismus, but with an anomaly of the position of rest or basic deviation. (The congenital strabismus syndrome is discussed separately.) Here we are talking about an acquired type of strabismus. Our discussion of heterophoria has shown that the physiologic position of rest is usually not parallel. In infants, it is often convergent. As a result, with poor fusion or breaking up of fusion, manifest convergence strabismus develops independent of the refractive error, specifically hyperopia. This is clearly demonstrated in secondary strabismus with unilateral loss of vision early in life, which generally results in esotropia, even without significant hyperopia.

The etiology of this convergence position of rest in infants is little understood. Most probably, it is the result of an increased convergence tone. It is not known if this increased convergence tone is caused by the central nervous system or if it relates to the fact that the medial recti have an innervation that is double that of the lateral recti. That the medial recti are innervated by version and vergence movement is demonstrated by the fact that they follow Hering's law for horizontal gaze but also have an opposite innervation in convergence. This is confirmed by the findings of Goldschmidt, which show that the number of nerve fiber endings in the medial rectus muscle is twice that of the lateral rectus for similar muscle-fiber types. It has been shown that the medial rectus muscle is represented at three places in the oculomotor nerve nucleus. One part is made up exclusively of nerve nuclei, which using retrograde tracer substances injected into the orbit are shown to be directed exclusively at the medial rectus muscle. These motor neurons are responsible for tonic functions. For this reason, there is a decrease in convergence in children treated with antiepileptic medications. Young monocular aphakics frequently lose their accommodative convergence. All these observations delineate the various ways that the convergent position of rest may be influenced.

With older children and adults, the motor position of rest is usually divergent. At this age, in secondary strabismus an aphakic or blind eye generally deviates outward.

This is readily seen in our patient population. Of children with divergence strabismus, three per cent have organic fundus changes or media opacities. In adults, this secondary strabismus rises to 12.3%. With convergence strabismus, 2.5% of children and 2.8% of adults showed organic fundus changes or medial opacities in the deviating eye.

Sensory mechanisms also play a role in the variation in degree or type of strabismus. If manifest strabismus develops for any cause with a normal sensory mechanism, it is accompanied by bothersome diplopia. These double images are more disturbing the closer they are to each other and the smaller the degree of deviation. In esotropia when the fusion mechanism for overcoming double vision is no longer adequate, the convergence mechanism is brought into play to eliminate double images at near gaze. The angle of deviation increases, and with it the distance between the double images. In this way, the diplopia becomes less bothersome. In this instance, one speaks of diplopia phobia (Van der Hoeve) or escape strabismus.[46]

Another possible means of overcoming the sensory disturbances is the blind-spot mechanism described by Swan. The disruptive second image disappears when it falls on the blind spot of the deviating eye. In fact, one finds a number of strabismic patients with a deviation of 15 degrees in whom the blind spot in the deviating eye forms the center of the zero point scotoma, or in whom the zero point scotoma is enlarged by inclusion of the blind spot.[132]

Differentiation of essential strabismus from accommodative strabismus occurs primarily by determining the refractive error and correcting it. If no hyperopia is present, the deviation must be viewed as essential — in other words, caused by the position of rest. If hyperopia is present and glasses correct the deviation, the diagnosis is made. If hyperopia is corrected with glasses and a manifest residual deviation exists with distance testing, then the corrected portion is accommodative and the residual deviation is essential. One also speaks of a basic deviation that remains after the accommodative elements have been eliminated through correction.

These considerations may appear labored. In practice, however, such differentiations are readily done by every ophthalmologist, in that surgery is performed on the essential strabismus or basic deviation. The basic deviation may be represented graphically on the abscissa, with divergence to the left of zero and the convergence position of rest to the right of zero.

The therapy for this type of strabismus follows from its description. Correction of a basic deviation can only be done by the prescription of prisms or, with larger deviations, surgery.

A classic example is the essential or acute strabismus of Franceschetti seen in adults. This is a sudden-onset convergent strabismus without hyperopia or evidence of muscle paresis (see section on acute strabismus).

In children, there is an acute form of strabismus analogous to that of the Franceschetti type which we call essential normosensorial late-onset strabismus. We discovered this type of strabismus while critically reviewing our results of therapy.[88]

We were interested in which types of strabismus were totally straight in free space following surgery. It turned out that this was true only for those cases of strabismus that first developed suddenly around age two to four years. For a short period of time, the strabismus is intermittent. Some children spontaneously admit to diplopia. This disappears after a few days, however, with a marked increase in the angle of deviation. Other children do not recognize the diplopia but, for the first few days after the onset of the deviation, close one eye. This eliminates bothersome double vision. Hyperopia or convergence excess is not present, and the angle cannot be eliminated by full correction of hyperopia. Typically, the angle of deviation increases over several months to about 25 degrees, sometimes more. The deviation is frequently alternating. Binocular examination sometimes shows normal correspondence and at other times shows suppression. The deviation often occurs early in the morning or after an afternoon nap and disappears one to two hours later. With an accommodative component, the deviation occurs more frequently at night and when the patient is tired.

The history of onset and its course are most characteristic. The two-pencil touch test is difficult because these children have lost binocularity. They act insecure and irritated; sometimes the parents feel that the child is crossing his eyes on purpose when he is upset. In fact, the child is upset because his eyes are crossed and suffers because of this. One has to consider esotropia secondary to increased intracranial pressure in the differential diagnosis. One must make it a rule always to look for papilledema in these cases.

Important therapeutic consequences result. In cases of normal sensory late-onset esotropia, one should not delay the surgery more than six months after onset of the deviation. In many of these cases, full return to parallelism of the eyes with normal bifoveal fixation can be achieved with surgery without use of intensive orthoptic exercises.

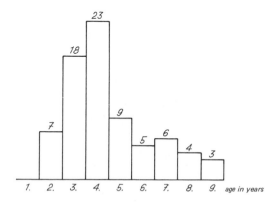

Fig. 48–Onset of strabismus in 75 cases of surgically fully cured esotropia. We are dealing primarily with normosensorial late-onset esotropia.

If surgery is delayed long periods of time, for example years, one may find that despite surgery, prismatic correction, and orthoptic exercises, a full return to normal binocular vision is no longer possible. It seems that after a prolonged period of time, suppression becomes deep seated, and "horror fusionis" no longer allows fusion at zero degrees. Even if one sets the eyes exactly on zero surgically or prismatically, one eye always deviates slightly to the side, down, or up. It dances around the parallel position without settling at orthotropia, which these cases usually do spontaneously after surgery.

It must be assumed that children younger than the age of two to two and one-half have a similar essential normal sensory strabismus. At this age, however, the sensory conditions are so labile and their adaptation to the deviation is so rapid that anomalous retinal correspondence or deep suppression with amblyopia develops. The chances of avoiding this sensory anomaly and restoring functional bifoveal vision are very low in such early-onset cases.

Normosensorial late-onset strabismus represents no more than 5% of all cases of esotropia. This diagnosis is important because therapy should not be delayed. One is dealing with a prognostically good type of strabismus. Proper therapy helps these patients optimally, but incorrectly handled, they are very unhappy people. This type of strabismus is not well known, in part because of the general reluctance to admit that total cures are so infrequent. This type of strabismus must be looked for among the entire patient population treated with any therapeutic method. Often, favorable results are reported with particular therapies, for example, prisms, binocular training, and so forth. These favorable results may be based on a biased patient selection or on the type of cases for which the therapies have been used. Cyclic strabismus also belongs in the group of types of normosensorial late-onset strabismus. Over time, these usually evolve into constant strabismus and require surgery. Here, too, the prognosis is favorable. In 1903, Worth wrote, "I have notes of a few cases which may properly be called periodic squints, in which the deviation has appeared every alternate day as regularly as a tertina ague."

These cases are rare; we have seen only a few ourselves. We have one patient who, following surgery for intermittent esotropia, developed an alternate-day convergence strabismus. We interpret these cases to be decompensation of the convergent position of rest. Psychologic factors are presumed to be partly responsible for the periodicity.

ACCOMMODATIVE STRABISMUS

Donders in 1864 was the first to show that convergence strabismus resulted from hyperopia.[45] Accommodation and convergence are linked. Hypermetropia requires increased accommodation and is accompanied by increased convergence, leading to esotropia.

Hypermetropia, along with convergence, has been subdivided by Donders into absolute, relative, and facultative types. With absolute hypermetropia, images cannot be focused on the retina, even with maximal effort. With relative hyperopia, adequate accommodation can be achieved only when convergence is used excessively, resulting in esotropia. If adequate accommodation can be achieved without convergence, then this hyperopia is called facultative.

This classification must be separated from the division of hyperopia into latent and manifest types, which together constitute total hyperopia. The latent portion of hyperopia manifests only after cycloplegia. Recognition of this has led to successful treatment of accommodative esotropia with full correction of the hyperopia using glasses.

The significance of hyperopia, specifically accommodation, for the strabismic process is unquestioned. To what degree this mechanism is responsible for convergent strabismus is debatable. There are hyperopes who never squint, and there are esotropes who are not hyperopic. Donders himself assumed that along with hyperopia, other factors — for example, loss of vision in one eye — had to be present for strabismus to develop. In our patient population, fully accommodative strabismus represents only 5% of esotropia. Partially accommodative strabismus is the most common form of esotropia. The individual concepts and mechanisms that play a role in accommodative strabismus were discussed previously.

Clinically, accommodative strabismus can be subdivided into four types and represented graphically on the Donders diagram.

FULLY ACCOMMODATIVE STRABISMUS WITH NORMAL AC/A RATIO

For simplicity's sake, it can be assumed that one diopter of accommodation is accompanied by one meter angle of convergence. With hyperopia of five diopters, five diopters of accommodation is needed to see clearly at a distance. For an object at 33 centimeters, eight diopters must be exerted. Without correction, this would lead to a convergence excess of five meter angles or 25 diopters with an interpupillary distance of five centimeters. This angle of deviation is eliminated both at distance and at near gaze with use of +5.00 diopter glasses. Diagnosis of fully accommodative strabismus is determined therapeutically. If the eyes are straight at distance and near gaze after full correction, this is fully accommodative strabismus. One further differentiation should be made. Only if the eyes remain straight on the alternate cover test is fully accommodative strabismus actually present. This is rarely the case. More commonly, the alternate cover test will reveal esophoria which is held straight by fusion. Under certain circumstances, surgery for esophoria is indicated.

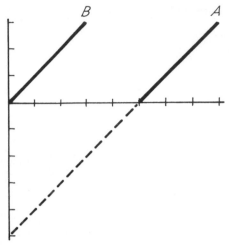

Fig. 49–Fully accommodative strabismus. Parallelism for distance and near gaze, esotropia with hyperopia of +5.
a) Without correction; and
b) With +5D correction.

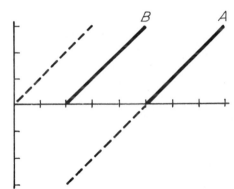

Fig. 50–Partially accommodative strabismic esotropia with hyperopia of +3.00 diopters.
a) Without correction; and
b) With glasses correction of +3.00. (There is a residual deviation of 2 meter angles.)

PARTIALLY ACCOMMODATIVE STRABISMUS WITH NORMAL AC/A RATIO

In this case, the angle of deviation is markedly reduced with use of glasses but manifest deviation remains, which is the same for distance and near gaze.

Theoretically, this residual angle must be eliminated through use of prisms or with surgery. In practice, however, it is very common for partially accommodative strabismus to differ sensorially from fully accommodative strabismus. Normal retinal correspondence is usually the rule with fully accommodative strabismus. With partially accommodative strabismus, the residual angle is maintained by abnormal retinal correspondence. These cases are extremely common. After correction of the hyperopia, numerous patients demonstrate microstrabismus. If orthotropia is present for distance with esophoria, one can operate. One performs either a bimedial rectus muscle recession or a resection of the lateral rectus and recession of the medial rectus on one eye. Some authors favor the retroequatorial myopexy (Faden operation, posterior fixation suture).

FULLY ACCOMMODATIVE STRABISMUS WITH RESIDUAL ANGLE FOR NEAR GAZE

In this condition, one is dealing with an abnormal relationship between accommodation and convergence, with convergence excess. With full correction of the hyperopia, the eyes are straight at distance but continue to be esotropic for near gaze. Usually, these patients are markedly hyperopic. The residual angle at near gaze must be corrected with bifocals or miotics.

PARTIALLY ACCOMMODATIVE STRABISMUS WITH CONVERGENCE EXCESS

With correction, the amount of deviation is reduced but a residual angle remains, which is greater at near gaze than at distance. To diagnose convergence excess or a high AC/A ratio, there should be an angle that is at least 10 diopters greater at near gaze than at distance. Theoretically, one should correct the residual deviation with use of prisms or surgery and the convergence excess with use of bifocals or miotics. Since anomalous retinal correspondence is usually present, the situation has to be viewed from a cosmetic aspect. As rational as all these considerations sound, carrying them out in practice is complicated. One has only to think of difficult cases in which, despite full optical correction and transient parallelism, the deviation has recurred and increased. There is a difference of opinion about the basic pathogenesis of accommodative strabismus and its relationship to refraction in the early years of life.

Numerous textbooks claim that hyperopia is greatest at birth and then declines from year to year. As a result of this, one can continuously decrease the strength of the correction. Other authors believe that hyperopia increases up to about eight years of age. We ourselves have observed that from year to year, we must increase the strength of the hyperopic correction.

Since the interpupillary distance increases with growth, convergence requirements increase and the convergence excess should decrease. Longitudinal studies have not been done concerning this point and the "outgrowing" of accommodative esotropia, however. There is a difference of opinion whether one can influence convergence excess surgically as well and whether treatment with miotics, bifocals, or penalization changes the convergence

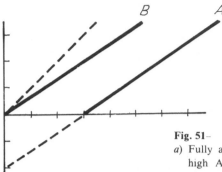

a)

Fig. 51–

a) Fully accommodative strabismus with a high AC/A ratio. Hyperopia of +2.00 diopters with convergence excess (high AC/A ratio). With +2.00 diopters, parallel for distance with a residual angle of 1.5 meter angles at 33 centimeters.

b) Bifocals in fully accommodative esotropia with convergence excess.

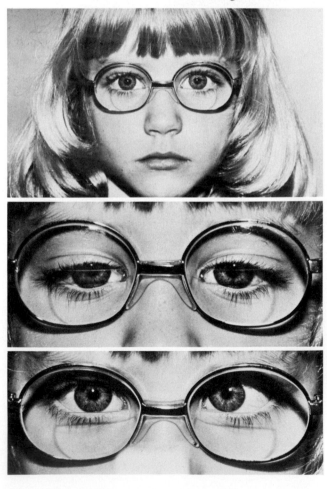

b)

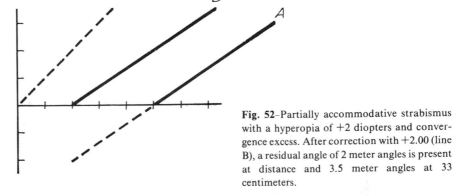

Fig. 52–Partially accommodative strabismus with a hyperopia of +2 diopters and convergence excess. After correction with +2.00 (line B), a residual angle of 2 meter angles is present at distance and 3.5 meter angles at 33 centimeters.

excess transiently or permanently. It is understood that in all cases, one has to prescribe glasses. Usually, one has to correct the total amount of hypertropia. In certain cases, however, one can choose to reduce the correction to that amount which provides orthotropia at near gaze and at distance.

It becomes difficult when one wishes to decrease the strength of the glasses or eliminate glasses entirely. Contact lenses are not always ideal. One has to consider that young people want to be without glasses at the swimming pool or at home in their own bedrooms without immediately manifest strabismus even when not using their hyperopic correction. In certain cases, on removing the glasses one can practice not accommodating and thereby converging. Vision is blurred in that situation, but there is no strabismus.

A high AC/A ratio or convergence excess may have two causes. In the *hypoaccommodative* type, a deficient accommodative system requires increased accommodative impulses. This results in excess convergence owing to the relationship between accommodation and convergence.

With the *hyperkinetic* type, accommodation is normal, but the convergence tone is increased. Each normal accommodative impulse is accompanied by excess convergence.

MICROTROPIA

In microtropia, we are dealing with a type of strabismus that is cosmetically not significant but plays an important role in our understanding of strabismus and amblyopia. By microtropia, we mean a cosmetic strabismus of less than five degrees with harmonious anomalous retinal correspondence.

The term "microtropia" was first proposed by us at the First International Strabismus Symposium in Giessen in 1966.[85] Up to that point, a variety of terms had been used in the literature, such as "small angle," "minimal anomaly," "inapparent strabismus," "retinal slip," "cortical slip," and, above all, "fixation disparity." The term "fixation disparity," however, had already been used by Ogle for a physiologic disparity within Panum's area with a maximum deviation of 20 minutes of arc.[109]

To avoid this misuse, Parks proposed the term "monofixational phoria."[112] We disagree with this term, since in this condition we are dealing with manifest strabismus — in other words, a tropia and not a phoria. Parks no longer speaks of monofixational phoria but uses the term "monofixation syndrome."[113] Included are not only anomalies with a manifest deviation but also those with parallelism and stereoamblyopia, amblyopia with anisometropia, and amblyopia of organic etiology. The term "syndrome" implies the occurrence of seemingly independent symptoms, appearing with each other, to create a specific entity. In this sense, the term "syndrome" does not apply to monofixation syndrome, since we are dealing with a symptom (suppression) that may occur with a variety of clearly defined clinical conditions.

Helveston and Von Noordon adopted the term "microtropia," but at first applied it only to cases in which the eccentric area used for fixation by the microtropic eye was "identical" with the binocular center of anomaly or zero point.[61]

In microtropia, binocular vision is based on harmonious anomalous retinal correspondence. Functionally, this is very important, since it provides depth perception and fusional movements. Stereopsis up to 40 seconds of arc on contour tests (not random dot) may be seen in very favorable cases. On the random-dot stereo test, however, stereopsis is markedly worse. The angle of deviation is so small that one would expect that orthotropia could be achieved with fusion, as occurs with heterophoria. The small angle of deviation is maintained through anomalous retinal correspondence, however, and resists prism therapy. Microtropia is almost always unilateral, and it is usually esotropic.

Microtropic amblyopia may vary in degree. In extreme cases, it is deep, with a dense central scotoma and eccentric fixation. Often, it is more moderate, with visual acuity of .5 (20/40) to .8 (20/25) and central fixation. The characteristics and significance of amblyopia with microtropia were discussed previously.

Based on fixation behavior, one can differentiate three types of microtropia.[83]

1. Cases with central fixation.
2. Cases with eccentric fixation. In this instance, the point of eccentric fixation is usually on a straight line between the fovea and the localization center of anomalous retinal correspondence.
3. In rare cases, the point of eccentric fixation and the center of localization for anomalous retinal correspondence (zero point) coincide. They are "identical."

One can differentiate between constant primary, primary decompensating, and secondary or consecutive microtropia.

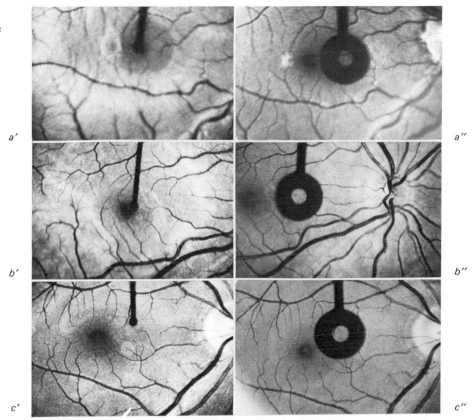

Fig. 53–Relationship between fixation and correspondence: in left-hand photos *a*, *b*, and *c*, the patient was asked to fixate on the target. The left eye was occluded. These photos show the monocular fixation. *a*, *b*, and *c* on the right show the localization center for abnormal retinal correspondence or zero point. The ring was perceived to be in the same direction as the fixation light seen with the other eye.[92] *a*) Microtropia with central fixation; *b*) Microtropia with eccentric fixation; and *c*) Microtropia with eccentric "identical" fixation.

Cases of primary microtropia have never had a larger angle of deviation. Acuity testing in infancy or in the first grade reveals unilateral vision loss. Sometimes amblyopia is first discovered in adulthood and must then be differentiated from organic amblyopia, specifically that with a neurologic basis. Primary microtropia may remain constant throughout life. We estimate constant primary microtropia to represent 0.9% to 1% of the entire population. Characteristically, these cases do not show any further heterophoria on the alternate cover test or show it only minimally. This strabismus is based primarily on a sensory disturbance, that is, on retinal correspondence that maintains a small stable angle of deviation.

Primary decompensating microtropia helps us understand the strabismic process. These are cases that decompensate into a larger angle of deviation in the first years of life. This occurs mainly when hyperopia, a convergent position of rest, or convergence excess or amblyopia coexist with microstrabismus. If we keep in mind that these factors by themselves can lead to convergent strabismus in the presence of normal binocularity, it is easy to understand why anisometropic amblyopia is more commonly seen without microtropia. Quite typical of this are children who begin to squint monocularly at the age of one to three years with a gradual increase in the angle without apparent subjective disturbances such as diplopia. Following full correction of hyperopia or elimination of amblyopia, the angle of deviation seems to disappear, but careful investigation reveals a small residual angle. These cases can be observed only when the children are brought very early for ophthalmic treatment.

In this case, one can assume that therapy leads to return to the status quo, that is, a pre-existing small angle. Important to this concept is the fact that the previously existing anomalous retinal correspondence is able to adapt to the variation in the angle better than in cases in which normal retinal correspondence was present at the onset. Familial cases also speak in favor of this concept. Patients without hypermetropia may show constant microtropia, while those with hypermetropia decompensate to a larger angle. In our judgment, 40% of all esotropias are caused by this decompensation. In these situations, we are usually dealing with matters of probability, since actual proof is lacking. It is useful to remember that cases of primary alternating strabismus do not fall into this group.

Besides cases of decompensated esotropia, there are also forms of microtropia that evolve into a divergent angle. Transitional cases exist. For example, convergent microtropia is present at near gaze with manifest divergence at distance. We believe that exotropia with amblyopia (which is usually rare with divergent strabismus) originally was microtropia.

Consecutive microtropia results after reduction of a larger angle, particularly following intensive orthoptics. It would be difficult in any specific case to decide whether one is dealing with primary decompensated or true secondary microtropia. The clinical history is definitive. The clinical findings

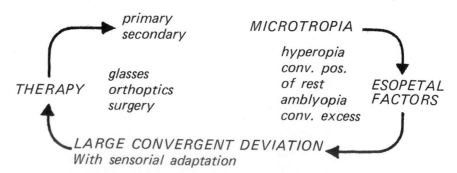

Fig. 54–The course of esotropic microtropia.

do not differ significantly between primary and consecutive microtropia. Consecutive microtropia usually has a larger additional heterophoria than does the primary type.

Refraction with microtropia frequently shows anisometropia if the microtropic eye is more hyperopic or has astigmatism. Marked anisometropia correlates with greater degrees of amblyopia. Often with eccentric fixation, microtropia may be secondary to astigmatism. The greater the degree of anisometropia, the poorer the prognosis for the amblyopia. With unilateral astigmatism, one is generally dealing with an anatomic anomaly. The spheric components of the anisometropia may be anatomically determined but may also occur owing to failure of emmetropization of the amblyopic eye. We have seen cases in which both eyes were equally hyperopic at approximately age nine. At age fourteen, the microtropic eye continued to show hyperopia, while the leading eye had become emmetropic.

Microstrabismus may appear together with heterophoria. Esophoria is especially common in secondary microtropia. It is this esophoria which for such a long time led to the lack of observation of the small manifest deviations.

The heredity of microtropia is particularly interesting. Primary microtropia appears to be determined by a hereditary factor. One frequently sees it clustered in families. At times, it is only primary microtropia; at other times it evolves into a larger angle of deviation. The amblyopia may be variable. The disposition to anomalous retinal correspondence appears to be inherited, but that for amblyopia is not.[89] We have been unable to differentiate whether this heredity is unifactorial or multifactorial.

Two methods are particularly useful in diagnosing microtropia: the unilateral cover test and the bifoveal correspondence test of Cüppers. Primarily, the diagnosis is made from the small refixation movements seen on the unilateral cover test. The alternate cover test shows additional heterophoria. The uncover test shows a fusional divergence movement that ends not in parallelism but in microtropia. Measurement of the manifest deviation is done with the simultaneous prism cover test, and the additional phoria deviation is measured with the alternate prism cover test. The angle of deviation may be judged by comparing the refixation movement with the Maddox cross.

Microtropia can be demonstrated photographically. With microtropia, the fourth Purkinje image is displaced nasally compared with the first Purkinje image of a microtropic eye.

If eccentric fixation is present with a cosmetically unapparent deviation, the diagnosis of microtropia is assured. This is true even with a negative mono- or unilateral cover test, since anomalous retinal correspondence is, so to speak, always present with eccentric fixation.

Anomalous retinal correspondence is best demonstrated ophthalmoscopically with the bifoveal correspondence test of Cüppers. It is often easier to show the angle of anomaly than the center of correspondence, since a suppression scotoma is often present in the region of the latter. Photographic representation of anomalous retinal correspondence is shown here. With Bagolini striated lenses, a small central gap is often seen in the light streak. This is an expression of the fixation point scotoma. This zero point scotoma may also be demonstrated with the binocular Amsler grid.

At the synoptophore, normal fusional ranges and stereopsis are often measured, leading the uninitiated to overlook the microtropia. However, if very small targets are used, although the subjective angle is at zero, the objective angle may be +2 or +3 degrees. If amblyopia is minimal, fusional ranges of +15 to –6 degrees may be measured at the synoptophore. Titmus stereo vision up to 40 seconds of arc may also be obtained. With the random-dot stereo test, however, stereopsis is markedly worse.

Heterophoria has to be considered in the differential diagnosis of microtropia. Microstrabismic amblyopia must be carefully differentiated from anisometropic amblyopia or amblyopia with discrete organic findings. Microstrabismus is usually not associated with anisometropia. Consequently, anisometropic amblyopia is more commonly seen without microtropia.

There are several theories regarding the pathogenesis of microtropia. Many authors consider microtropia the result of heterophoria. This heterophoria leads to suppression in the macular region and to expansion of the surrounding Panum's area with a subsequent change in correspondence.

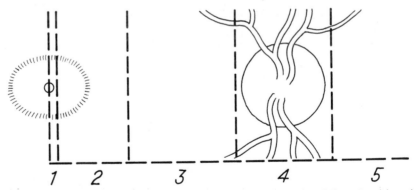

Fig. 55–Classification according to the extent of deviation. 1. Anomalies of binocular vision with parallelism up to 0.5 degrees. 2. Microtropia of 0.5 to 5 degrees. 3. Small angle strabismus of 5 to 12 degrees. 4. Blind spot mechanism of 12 to 18 degrees. 5. Large angle deviation of greater than 18 degrees (large angle strabismus).

According to Helveston and von Noorden, microtropia results from anisometropia.[61] This causes a central scotoma leading to eccentric fixation. Around this eccentric fixation anomalous retinal correspondence develops. We feel that microtropia is present primarily as a sensory anomaly.

In the discussion on the mechanisms of fixation and fusion, Goldman concluded for theoretic reasons that there must be a statistical variant in the interaction of the feedback mechanism whereby a small angle with intact fusion and stereopsis develops.[55] Our numerous observations of cases of primary microtropia support this viewpoint.

Richter, in an investigation of the heredity of strabismus, found several families with inherited sensory anomalies equivalent to our microtropia.[122] Independently we have drawn attention to the hereditary factor in microtropia.[86] Holland made similar observations.[67]

The therapy for microtropia consists primarily of the treatment of amblyopia. This usually responds well to occlusion. Once vision has recovered adequately, we start graded occlusion using press-on filters of decreasing intensity (Bangerter's filters). We occlude each eye alternately until the child is able to read fluently with either eye and until alternation occurs freely with an occlusion filter density of one (weakest). In our experiences, this usually requires treatment up to the age of ten years. Even with this method of treatment, spontaneous alternation does not develop with microtropia.

Anomalous retinal correspondence appears to be refractory to treatment. After the above-named therapy, one usually achieves harmonious anomalous retinal correspondence with a fair degree of binocular vision and without asthenopic symptoms. In rare cases, full parallelism with normal binocular vision results. Even in these cases, however, it is better if one remains skeptical and treats further with occlusion filters as if microtropia was present. Much too often, one sees a significant problem with reading in adults with microtropia who have normal distance acuity. This should be prevented by use of the graded occlusion just outlined.

If in addition there is a latent component to the deviation, especially if microtropia shows signs of decompensation, the excess deviation should be treated surgically. One can correct the extra heterophoria with use of prisms prior to surgery. Sometimes recession of one medial rectus is adequate; more often, however, a small recession resection is necessary. The treatment of these is like that of heterophorias.

In our patient population of 33,000, microtropia was found in 2.84%, primary constant strabismus in 1.34%. Among esotropes, microtropia represented 40%. Of these, 20% were primary constant microtropia and a further 20% primary decompensated or secondary microtropia. Of all exotropias, divergent microtropia represented only 3.6%. The percentage in adults is 4.8% and therefore considerably higher than in children, at 1.6%.[94]

THE CONGENITAL STRABISMUS SYNDROME

The term "congenital strabismus" implies that strabismus was present at birth. There is, however, a uniform opinion that "congenital strabismus"

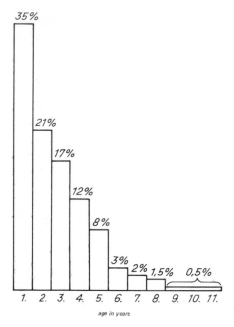

Fig. 56–Onset of strabismus in 600 children with esotropia: ages and years.

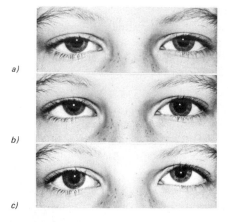

Fig. 57–Dissociated vertical deviation, or alternating hypertropia with congenital strabismus.

a) Nearly parallel;
b) Hypertropia of right eye after occlusion of right eye; and
c) Hypertropia of left eye after occlusion of left eye.

should include not only strabismus present since birth but also that with an onset in the first few months of life. One can actually speak of a congenital strabismus syndrome. It is a judgment question whether one requires strabismus to be present in the first three months, the first four months, or, according to Constenbater, in the first six months of life. Since the fovea is not fully developed until the fourth month of life, this time period seems natural to us. The term "infantile esotropia" implies that strabismus develops during infancy—in other words, during the first year of life.

It is not surprising that strabismus present since birth has different characteristics from that which develops in the second year of life. Careful observation over the years has shown us that children whose strabismus was present in the first few months of life have a very characteristic type of strabismus.[87] The various symptoms are present in this type of deviation in certain percentages.

— dissociated vertical divergence	90% of cases
— latent nystagmus	55% of cases
— head tilt	70% of cases
— torsion	65% of cases

With dissociated vertical divergence, the nonfixing eye is higher or deviates up under the cover. This phenomenon is best observed by viewing the eye behind the cover. On removing the cover, the eye spontaneously returns to, but never quite reaches, vertical alignment.

Dissociated vertical divergence movements can also be observed in the nonfixing eye when one places a neutral density filter or red glass in front of the fixing eye. The nonfixing eye makes a downward movement and returns to straight ahead as soon as the dark glass is removed. This is called the Bielschowsky phenomenon. Dissociated vertical divergence appears to have a central nervous system innervational mechanism. It is to be separated from strabismus sursoadductorius (overacting inferior oblique), which has a peripheral muscular etiology.

Latent nystagmus is a jerk nystagmus with the rapid phase aimed in the direction of the fixing eye. When both eyes are open, the eyes are quiet; on covering one eye, the nystagmus develops. Spontaneous vertical or rotary nystagmus also occurs along with horizontal jerk nystagmus. This nystagmus

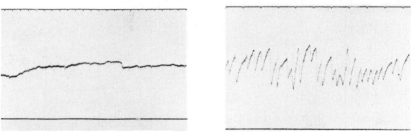

a) Quiet eye position with both eyes open;   b) Nystagmus, rapid phase left, after covering the right eye; and

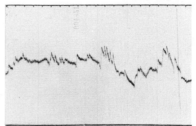

c) Nystagmus, rapid phase right, after covering the left eye.

Fig. 58–Electrooculographic demonstration of latent nystagmus.

can be readily seen at the slit lamp or with the ophthalmoscope. Sometimes nystagmus is present with both eyes open. The rapid phase is then always aimed in the direction of the dominant eye. On covering the nondominant eye, the nystagmus naturally increases in amplitude. One speaks of manifest latent nystagmus. Usually, amplitude is greater and most easily seen in the nondominant eye. When a deeply amblyopic eye is forced to fixate, the slow and rapid phase of the nystagmus slows down to a slow-motion-type tempo.

A head tilt is common in congenital strabismus; this has to be differentiated from ocular torticollis. The cause of this head tilt is not clear, but it is not a mechanism to avoid diplopia.

Infants with cerebral damage frequently lift their chin, tilting their head backwards. Similarly, small children often tilt the head to the side of the fixing eye. Typically this is crossfixation; in other words, left gaze is done with the right eye fixing and the face turned right, and on right gaze the face turns left and fixation is with the left eye. Exotropia occasionally behaves oppositely—the right eye fixes on right gaze and the left eye on left gaze. The face in this situation is turned in the opposite direction.

In older children and adults, the head is often tilted toward one shoulder. This is usually the shoulder on the side of the fixing eye. This head position can be provoked in some patients. For example, to test vision in the right eye, the left eye is covered, and there is an involuntary head tilt toward the right shoulder. This head tilt reverses on testing the left eye and covering the right.

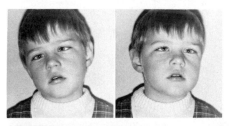

Fig. 59–Head tilt in congenital esotropia.
a) Right fixation: head is to the right shoulder, face to the right; and
b) Left fixation: head is to the left shoulder, face left.

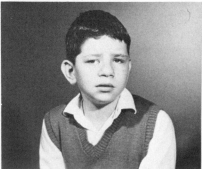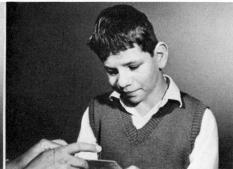

Fig. 60–Head tilt in congenital esotropia with Little's disease. *a*) Distance vision: right eye fixing, face to the left, head to the left shoulder; and *b*) Near vision: left eye fixing, face right, head to the right shoulder.

In rare cases, the exact opposite is true—the head is tilted to the side of the fixing eye.

The fourth phenomenon of the congenital strabismus syndrome is torsion, which is seen with careful observation of the iris. The eye that picks up fixation makes an inward torsional movement, while the eye giving up fixation rotates outward. This is true even when the eye picking up fixation is hypotropic.

The angle of deviation varies greatly in congenital esotropia. Well known are those cases in which the eyes are virtually fixed at an angle of 40 to 45 degrees. This is referred to as "strabismus fixus." These cases mimic bilateral abducens paresis. Only after occlusion, after surgery, or spontaneously in the first year of life does it become obvious that abduction is possible past the midline and that abducens paresis is not present. Mechanical factors may be primarily responsible for these cases of maximal adduction. Some authors believe that blockage of nystagmus by convergence is the cause of the esotropia.

In most children, the angle of deviation is unstable and highly variable, related to fatigue, the psychic condition, and so forth. Sometimes one can see fusional divergence movements that never quite reach parallelism. "A–" patterns are as common in congenital strabismus as "V–" patterns.

With accommodative influences, the angle of deviation may increase during the first years of life. Occasionally, there is a spontaneous decrease in the angle, and in rare cases a spontaneous consecutive divergence may even result. Strabismus associated with cerebral palsy is not uncommonly divergent or, if convergent, often becomes divergent over time.

Sometimes it is difficult to observe all these symptoms in infants. Specific symptoms such as dissociated vertical divergence are not as pronounced early in life as they are later. They become more obvious in the second year of life. The various symptoms mentioned that constitute the congenital strabismus syndrome can also be observed in adults. The entire clinical picture is so characteristic that the diagnosis can be made in a short period of time by simple observation.

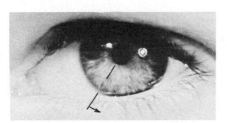 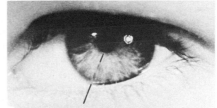

Fig. 61 A and B–Congenital strabismus: Incyclotorsion of the eye which picks up fixation (taken from a movie).

The pathogenesis and etiology of congenital strabismus are unclear. One should keep the following embryonal and early-childhood developmental changes in mind. The optical system, in contrast to the vestibular system, develops relatively late. The vestibular nerve is already fully myelinated in the sixth month of gestation. Minkowsky showed extension and flexion of extremities on a shift in position during the sixth month of gestation.[103] This indicates a functioning vestibular system at that time. In contrast, the optic nerve is not fully myelinated at birth, and the macula upon which fixation is dependent is not anatomically fully developed until the fourth month of life. If an error in the position of the eyes exists prior to the fourth month of life, this leads to difficulty with the coordination between optic and vestibular influences. We consider the previously mentioned symptoms, namely double dissociated vertical divergence, latent nystagmus, cyclotorsion, and head tilt, as proof of this.

Such disturbances can also result from cerebral lesions, for example, birth trauma. The evidence of this is the fact that cerebrally damaged children have a higher incidence of this type of strabismus.

Recently, we have developed another hypothesis to explain the congenital strabismus syndrome. We feel that it is a competition from the extra geniculostriate system.[87a] Beside the path from the retina to the lateral geniculate body, and from there to area 17, a variety of other pathways exist that do not go to the lateral geniculate body but instead go directly to the midbrain. Trevarthen and Sperry assume that this second pathway, which goes to the superior colliculus and to the pulvinar serves ambient vision. Twenty to 30% of optic nerve fibers do not end at the lateral geniculate. The majority of these are probably uncrossed fibers from the nasal retinal half. These represent phylogenetically and ontogenetically older pathways than the geniculostriate system. With prematurity, cerebral damage, or other causes, phylogenetically older systems may retain their predominance over the younger system. The nasal retinal halves and the ambient surrounding vision dominate foveal and direct discriminatory vision. Fixation is on the nasal side of both fovea, and the eyes assume a convergent position. Only with development does fixation return to the fovea, but it has a tendency to slide over to the nasal retinal half. When both eyes are open, these opposing tendencies of both eyes are balanced. When one eye is closed, this balance fails, and latent nystagmus manifests. This is only a hypothesis. It serves the purpose, however, of forcing one to think about the congenital strabismus syndrome and therapeutically reachable goals.

Birth traumas—specifically, asphyxia in the neonatal period, kernicterus, or orbital changes—must be considered as causes. Heredity plays a minimal role in this type of strabismus. Because of the vertical deviation, paralyses are often suspected. Lesions of the central nervous system rarely lead to the paresis of individual muscles; instead, they lead to abnormal coordination between innervation and muscle action. This is also true for the oculomotor muscles, and the abovementioned characteristics are less the results of isolated oculomotor paresis than an expression of difficulties in central nervous system coordination.

The differential diagnosis includes pseudostrabismus and intermittent strabismus in small children. If at age two a child with pseudostrabismus develops accommodative strabismus, the parents will undoubtedly swear the child has had strabismus since birth, with a late aggravation of the condition. Lack of the characteristic signs of congenital strabismus allows for clear differentiation.

Intermittent strabismus of the newborn consists of transient convergent spasms. In between the convergent episodes, both eyes are parallel, and normal binocular function can develop. Intermittent convergence spasms are not pathologic, and they disappear within the first half-year of life.

Even with the Duane's retraction syndrome, there are specific eye positions in which binocularity is present and the typical signs of congenital strabismus are usually absent.

In our experience, it is very rare that a child who has squinted since birth fails to show any of the abovementioned signs. Conversely, if the abovementioned symptoms are present, very early onset of the strabismus is most likely, even if the history does not clearly indicate this. The primary therapeutic goals are maintenance of alternation and cosmetic surgery. It is not surprising with such symptomatology and presumed etiology that complete cure of strabismus is not possible. The earlier one operates, the better the sensory results are supposed to be. However, even with late operations, we have achieved relatively good binocularity, as proven by the two-pencil touch test. Since early surgery is associated with problems in the control of amblyopia and subsequent late changes in the deviation, we do not feel that early surgery is mandatory. In our population, the congenital strabismus syndrome represents 15% of esotropes.

DIVERGENT STRABISMUS

Exotropia is less common than esotropia. In our clinical patient population, esotropia is four times as common as exotropia. In adults, it is two to one. In esotropia, children account for 52% of the total cases, whereas in exotropia adults predominate (56%). Fifty-eight per cent of child exotropes have intermittent deviation, whereas only 34% of adult exotropes are intermittent.

Microstrabismus is extremely rare in exotropia. Only 3.6% of our patients with exotropia have microstrabismus. There is a slightly higher incidence in adults (4.8%) than in children (1.6%).

There are children who spontaneously go from esotropia into exotropia. This is not common, however, and occurs spontaneously in only 1.5% of our children with esotropia.

INTERMITTENT EXOTROPIA

As the name implies, this is a strabismus that shows up only intermittently. Two types can be distinguished: Those that are intermittent for distance and those intermittent for near vision. Intermittent exotropia at distance is a typical clinical picture. On near gaze, the eyes are parallel, and one eye deviates out on distance fixation.

In mild cases, the deviation is seen only sporadically, for example, when the child is tired, daydreaming, or looking off into space. At the time of examination, one may have difficulty in finding the deviation as the child's alertness is aroused.

In marked cases, the divergence may be constant at distance, and even at near gaze the eyes may be held parallel only with great effort, such as when a very small object is presented for fixation.

Parents will frequently see the child close one eye in bright sunlight. This sign is almost pathognomonic for intermittent exotropia. Absence of this sign, however, does not speak against an intermittent exotropia.

In intermittent exotropia, there is an alternation between latent and manifest strabismus. The divergent position of rest is compensated for through fusion aided by voluntary and tonic convergence.

There is a significant difference between intermittent exotropia and intermittent esotropia. Esotropia can only be compensated for by fusion, not by voluntary divergence. For this reason, intermittent esotropia rapidly evolves into constant strabismus. The evolution that in exotropia takes months to years, occurs with esotropia in a matter of days to weeks.

Onset in most cases is in the first years of life, but its evolution can be highly variable. There are children who go through the phase of experiencing a manifest deviation for distance, with a few months of becoming constantly divergent for distance. After a few more months, they may even be exotropic

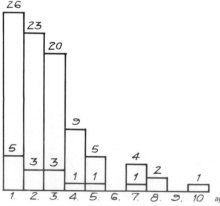

Fig. 62–Onset of strabismus in ninety children with exotropia.
1. Column base: constant exotropia; and
2. Remainder of the column: intermittent exotropia.

for near vision. Other children rarely manifest a deviation at distance and have no evidence of further deterioration.

Simple inspection or the unilateral cover test shows manifest deviation for distance and the parallel position at near gaze. The alternate cover test is important in bringing out the entire basic deviation. Two types of intermittent exotropia at distance exist.

In the most common type, the deviation is the same at distance and near gaze when measured with the alternate cover test. This type is called "basic exodeviation." In the position of rest, exotropia appears for distance and near vision, and the relationship of accommodation to convergence, the AC/A ratio, is normal. To this group also belong those cases in which the angle at near gaze at first appears smaller than at distance, even with the alternate cover test. However, after a short period (one hour) of occlusion of one eye to suspend fusion, the near angle increases to equal to or larger than what it is at distance. Burian coined the term "pseudodivergence excess" for these cases.[24] As shall be explained, one would do better to consider these cases as an exotropic position of rest with pseudoconvergence excess.

In rare cases, even after occlusion of one eye, the angle at near vision is considerably smaller than that at distance. In our opinion, this is a divergent position of rest with convergence excess and a high AC/A ratio. In these cases, relying on Duane's classification, Burian used the term "true divergence excess." This term implies that divergence is an active process. What one is actually measuring with the alternate cover test, however, is a true divergent position of rest at distance combined with convergence excess for near gaze.

Since normal binocular vision is present, at least intermittently, there is normal retinal correspondence which functions very well at near gaze. At distance, the deviating eye is suppressed, and in this situation a harmonious anomalous retinal correspondence is said to develop. It is claimed that normal retinal correspondence can then alternate with anomalous retinal correspondence according to the position of the eyes.

Significant amblyopia does not exist, specifically not in those cases that alternate. If the same eye is always the deviating eye it can become somewhat weaker than the other, but amblyopia never reaches the same depths as with esotropia.

At the synoptophore, objective measurements frequently show a surprisingly large angle of deviation. It is "surprisingly large" insofar as one would expect instrument convergence to give a smaller angle. The subjective answers vary according to the relationship between fusion and suppression. The angle of deviation is often larger with pictures seen simultaneously than with fusion or stereo pictures.

Often during divergence in intermittent exotropia, there is a vertical deviation of one eye. Usually the deviating eye is higher. It is generally not possible to demonstrate a true overaction or paresis of a vertical motor muscle. One gets the impression that this is similar to the double dissociated

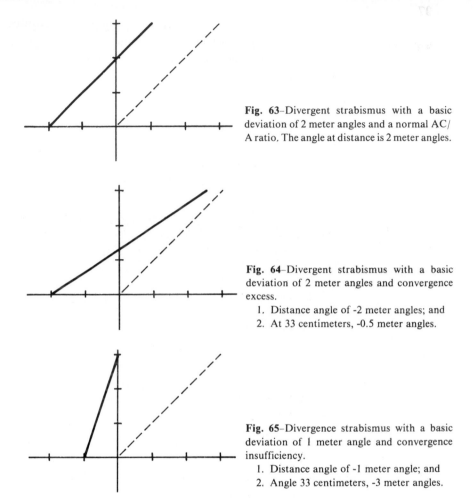

Fig. 63–Divergent strabismus with a basic deviation of 2 meter angles and a normal AC/A ratio. The angle at distance is 2 meter angles.

Fig. 64–Divergent strabismus with a basic deviation of 2 meter angles and convergence excess.
1. Distance angle of -2 meter angles; and
2. At 33 centimeters, -0.5 meter angles.

Fig. 65–Divergence strabismus with a basic deviation of 1 meter angle and convergence insufficiency.
1. Distance angle of -1 meter angle; and
2. Angle 33 centimeters, -3 meter angles.

vertical divergence in esotropia. Occasionally, however, the deviating eye will be depressed.

If there is an overaction of the oblique muscles, one can differentiate two types. Overaction of the inferior oblique gives a "V" pattern. In this case, the exotropia becomes manifest not only at distance but also on upgaze at near vision.

Superior oblique overaction results in an "A" pattern. The deviation is manifest primarily on downgaze. There is a simultaneous convergence insufficiency. Convergence is usually very good in intermittent exotropia except in those patients showing overaction of the superior obliques or with convergence insufficiency.

Uncorrected myopia can induce exophoria or increase an existing exophoria. Particularly unfavorable are cases of unilateral astigmatism or anisomyopia. In contrast, hyperopia counteracts the tendency toward divergence.

There is an intermittent exotropia in which the deviation is greater at near vision than at distance. The eyes are usually parallel for distance, but at near vision one eye deviates markedly. The difference between distance and near gaze should be at least 10 to 15 diopters. In these cases, one can speak of a convergence insufficiency or a low AC/A ratio. Frequently, there is a large interpupillary distance—specifically, hypertelorism. Patients with overaction of the superior oblique ("A" pattern) often belong to this category.

Intermittent exotropia is often familial. Some family members may show a very limited, others a highly developed, exodeviation. The direction of the tendency toward deviation seems to be inherited; the extent, however, can be variable.

Treatment must fit the findings, age, and clinical course. In general, it is surgical. If in a small child the eyes diverge, treatment is rarely necessary. Nonetheless, it is useful to encourage accommodation and convergence through use of small toys and near vision activities. If the eyes deviate frequently, the child should be alerted to this by the parents when it happens. The simple request to "look straight ahead" combined with voluntary blinking often allows the child to correct the deviation transiently. In this way, he obtains a subjective impression about the position of his eyes. When the eyes begin to show constant divergence, even at near gaze, surgery is indicated even in a small child.

Optical correction should be indicated in all cases in which myopia, anisometropia, or astigmatism is present. With hyperopia, use of a corrective prescription usually aggravates the exodeviation by relaxing accommodation. In certain situations, overcorrection of the myopia or prescription of concave glasses even with hyperopia may be indicated.

Orthoptic treatment is primarily directed against suppression. Awareness of physiologic diplopia and broadening of the fusional range help in compensating for this deviation tendency. When convergence is adequate, which is usually the case, convergence exercises are not needed. Practice with Bagolini striated glasses or looking at a point light source enables one to recognize the deviation subjectively and compensate for it by fusion. The two-pencil pointing test is also a useful exercise.

Surgery is usually unavoidable if the basic deviation is greater than 10 degrees (16 to 18 diopters). Basic exotropia has a tendency to increase during puberty and the growth spurt. The first operation at approximately age six may often have to be repeated at a later date.

The latest that surgery should be performed is when the patient becomes constantly exotropic at distance and near vision. It should not be deferred because further waiting would lead to marked suppression. Longstanding cases show horror fusionis. Our preferred surgery is a recession of a lateral rectus combined with resection of the medial rectus on the same eye. Certain authors prefer to operate on the dominant eye. To the parents and other authors, operation on the deviating eye would seem most logical. In cases in which the deviation is much less at near gaze than at distance, gaze recession of both lateral rectus muscles is indicated.

It is commonly claimed that it is impossible to overcorrect exotropia. This only seems to be true because most cases are markedly undercorrected surgically. Overcorrection can occur if the lateral rectus is recessed too much or if an existing hyperopia is ignored. If convergence exercises have been done, the patients almost always develop convergence spasms postoperatively, which lead to convergence excess esotropia. Postoperative diplopia should therefore not be allowed to remain but should be compensated for with base-out prisms. Usually, use of the prisms can gradually be reduced. It is wise to warn the parents about the possibility of the need for temporary postoperative prism glasses, the use of miotics, or the use of patching or plus lenses if hyperopia is present. Alternate occlusion and myopia can be employed with surgical overcorrection to avoid postoperative escape into convergence strabismus.

If one reexamines these patients after a number of years, one frequently has to operate again or take further measures to prevent recurrent divergence. Recently, preoperative compensation of the angle of deviation with prisms has been recommended. Appropriate controls, comparative studies assessing the value of this therapy, are lacking.

CONSTANT EXOTROPIA

As indicated previously, constant exotropia can be the end result of intermittent exotropia. In this case, one should differentiate between primary, secondary, and postoperative exotropia.

Cases of congenital exotropia do exist, especially in children with brain damage, and all the characteristics of congenital strabismus are present. Individuals with unilateral organic loss of vision or with functional amblyopia have a tendency to diverge, as in unilateral high myopia. If one finds functional amblyopia and anomalous retinal correspondence in exotropia, one should remember that primary microstrabismus may also become exotropic. Exotropia may occur more-or-less rapidly following surgical correction of esotropia. This may occur with extreme surgery or with postoperative restriction of the medial rectus muscle. If this occurs, even with careful measurement and surgical technique, one should remember that there are cases of esotropia that over a period of years spontaneously evolve to orthotropia or even become exotropic. If one operates on such cases, for which the prognosis is difficult to determine, the postoperative exotropia becomes understandable.

The treatment goal for constant exotropia that has evolved from intermittency as well as for exotropia associated with aphakia is functional. Parallelism with normal binocular vision should result after surgery.

Recession of the lateral rectus and resection of the medial rectus should not be so extensive as to produce a postoperative incomitance. In cases of undercorrection, prisms can be used, and the angle of deviation may spontaneously decrease further under the influence of fusion.

In all other cases, the goal of treatment is cosmetic. Severe deviations require significant surgery, which may include total tenotomy of the external rectus muscle. In all cases of constant exotropia, we perform the two-pencil touch test. Sometimes patients will return their eyes to orthotropia for this task. This is an indication that the deviation was originally intermittent and has a good prognosis.

"A" AND "V" PATTERNS

The concept of "concomitant strabismus" actually means that the angle of deviation is the same in all directions of gaze with either the right or the left eye fixing.

Duane described patients in whom the angle of strabismus was different on upgaze from that on downgaze.[47] More recently, Urrets-Zavalia, Urist, and Costenbader renewed interest in these cases.[31,134,135] The term "A" pattern derives from Jampolsky, "V" pattern from Albert.[75] The term "syndrome" has been allowed to lapse because not all preconditions have been met for this. One speaks of "A" and "V" patterns instead.

With "V" pattern esotropia, the angle is greater on downgaze than on upgaze. With exotropia, the angle of deviation is greater on upgaze. The difference between up- and downgaze should be at least 8 degrees or 15 diopters, with a difference in elevation and depression of 25 degrees.

In "A" pattern esotropia, the eyes are more convergent on upgaze than on downgaze. With exotropia, the exodeviation is greater on downgaze than on upgaze. The difference here should be 5 degrees or 10 prism diopters.[79]

Other symptoms may be added to this incomitance of the horizontal angle of deviation, depending upon the direction of vertical gaze. With "V" pattern, there is often elevation of the adducted eye (strabismus sursoadductorius); in other words, overaction of the inferior oblique muscle. Another sign that one often sees is an antimongoloid slant to the lid fissures; ie, a downward slant temporally. The eyes are often excyclorotated. One can determine this ophthalmoscopically by the position of the fovea versus the disc or perimetrically by the position of the blind spot.

With "A" patterns, there is often a strabismus deorsoadductorius; in other words, an overaction of the superior oblique. Lid fissures often are mongoloid. The eyes frequently are incyclorotated. The incidence of "A" and "V" patterns varies in the literature between 12.5% and 50%. This depends in part on the differences in methods of examination and the criteria applied. In our strabismus patient population, we found "A" patterns in 5.5% and "V" patterns in 7.5%, for a total of 13%. Within the congenital squint syndrome group, however, we found a 44% incidence of "A" and "V" patterns. Patients with hydrocephalus frequently have an "A" pattern.

There is little agreement regarding the etiology of "A" and "V" patterns. Four possible causes are discussed here.

1. The axis of excursion of the globes is not perfectly horizontal. In the "V" pattern it is higher nasally, and in the "A" pattern it is lower nasally, as if both orbits were tilted around the sagittal axis. This results in increased convergence on downgaze or upgaze and elevation or depression of the adducted eye. In the case of a "V" pattern, greater innervation has to reach the superior rectus on the right to keep the eye horizontal. This greater impulse is coupled to its contralateral synergist, the inferior oblique, resulting in elevation of the adducted left eye.

2. The strength of the vertical muscles is not fully balanced for side gaze. This is particularly true of the inferior and superior obliques.

   The investigations of Krewson showed that as a rule the elevating action of the inferior oblique is stronger than the depressing action of the superior oblique.[80] This imbalance has an anatomic cause. The axis along which the action takes place is more sagittal for the inferior oblique than for the superior oblique. In adduction, therefore, the inferior oblique reaches its elevating field of action before the superior oblique reaches its field of depression. This results in elevation of the adducted eye, which is especially evident on extreme adduction as occurs with unilateral large-angle strabismus.

3. Paresis of the superior oblique results in a "V" pattern. Whether this is associated with esotropia or exotropia depends upon the position of rest and the refractive status. Paresis of the inferior oblique results in an "A" pattern.

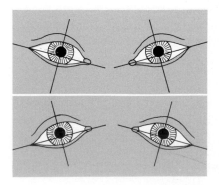

Fig. 66–

a) "A" pattern: marked convergence on upgaze, mongoloid lid slants, depression in adduction.

b) "V" pattern: marked divergence on upgaze, elevation in adduction, and antimongoloid lid slants.

4. One assumes that physiologically the medial recti have greater action on downgaze, and the lateral recti on upgaze. For this reason, Urist developed the hypothesis that in "V" esotropia the medial recti are overacting, and in "A" exotropia they are underacting. "V" exotropia results from overaction of the lateral recti, and "A" esotropia from underaction of the lateral recti.

To what degree other innervational disturbances, for example coinnervation, play a role in "A" and "V" patterns is difficult to determine. Electromyographic investigation in this regard fails to provide a definitive opinion. It is crucial, in our viewpoint, that "A" and "V" patterns inducing elevation or depression in adduction be differentiated from dissociated vertical deviations.

Elevation or depression in adduction is determined by anatomy or muscle paresis if the vertical action of the obliques is not perfectly balanced.

Dissociated vertical deviation or alternating sursumduction is determined by cerebral innervation. Elevation or depression in adduction can affect all types of strabismus whenever the angle of deviation is very large or the balance is markedly disturbed. Dissociated vertical divergence affects only congenital strabismus or that with onset in early infancy and can be combined with elevation or depression on adduction.

Besides the divergent and convergent "A" and "V" patterns, mixed forms exist. In the "V" patterns, the globes are convergent on downgaze, parallel for straight ahead, and divergent on upgaze. These cases are especially interesting because of their sensory adaptation. Normal binocular vision with normal retinal correspondence may be present in straight-ahead gaze. In the other directions of gaze, suppression or diplopia occurs. Those patients who maintain normal binocular vision through a head tilt are important—for example, those who look up and depress the chin with "V" esotropia.

"A" and "V" pattern strabismus, however, may reveal anomalous retinal correspondence of a harmonious type in which the angle of anomaly corresponds to the variable angle of deviation.

"A" and "V" patterns can be approached surgically. However, surgery is not necessary in all cases. It is especially indicated when binocular vision is maintained only by a head tilt or the strabismus is a cosmetically disturbing factor. Recommendations for the exact type of surgery vary greatly.

With purely horizontal "A" and "V" patterns, symmetric operation on the horizontally acting recti is recommended: for example, with "V" esotropia, a recession of both medial recti; with "A" esotropia, a resection of both lateral recti; with "V" exotropia, recession of both lateral recti; and with "A" exotropia, resection of both medial recti.[134]

If simultaneously there is overaction of the obliques, these should be weakened at the same time. For example, with "V" esotropia with overaction of both inferior obliques, both medial recti are recessed and the inferior obliques weakened by a recession or myectomy.[41,54]

Another surgical approach consists of vertically offsetting the insertion of the horizontal rectus muscles. With "V" esotropia, the recessed medial rectus should simultaneously be displaced inferiorly; in other words, to approximate the action of the inferior rectus. The adducting effect of the inferior rectus is weakened, and its pressor effect becomes manifest. In this way, the situation that exists on upgaze should be spread to downgaze. The reverse exists for "A" esotropia. With exotropia, the external rectus is recessed and displaced upward. With "A" exotropia, the external rectus on both sides is recessed and displaced downward.[79]

Other authors displace the vertical rectus muscles in a horizontal direction; for example, with "A" esotropia, the superior rectus is displaced temporally.[102]

More recently, an oblique recession or resection of the horizontal recti has been recommended. For example, with "V" esotropia, the medial rectus is recessed more inferiorly than superiorly; the reverse is done with "A" esotropia. The same procedure can be used with a combined recession resection. For example, with "V" esotropia, more recession of the medial rectus inferiorly and more resection of the lateral rectus inferiorly are done.[17,19,96] Our experience with this surgical method has not been satisfactory.

Besides the classic "A" and "V" patterns, more rare types occur, including "X," "Y," and lambda patterns.

ACUTE STRABISMUS

ACUTE ESOTROPIA OF BIELSCHOWSKY[15]

In myopes, it is not uncommon to find esotropia that begins late in life. Women are affected more often than men. It is characteristic of this clinical entity that esotropia is only present at distance. On near gaze, both eyes are straight or have minimal esophoria which can be compensated. Adduction is frequently limited.

The patients complain particularly about diplopia at distance but are free of symptoms at near gaze. Some patients do not suffer from diplopia even though they have a manifest deviation at distance with normal binocular vision at near gaze. Usually this is due to insufficient correction of the myopia, leading to blurred vision for distance and allowing suppression of one image to occur.

The etiology of this entity is not clear. It is possible that with preexisting esophoria and insufficient correction of the myopia, the fusional impulse is inadequate at distance as a result of the blurred vision, while it is maintained with clearer vision at near gaze. There are, however, transitional cases between the acute esotropia of Bielschowsky and the myopathy of severe myopes. Over a number of years, adduction of both eyes with limitation of movement may evolve out of this esotropia at distance. Some authors speak of a divergence paresis.

The therapy of choice is base-out prisms. One does not need to prescribe correction for the total amount of the deviation, but does need to use the minimal prism that still allows fusion. In advanced cases, surgery is necessary.

Acute strabismus of the Bielschowsky type is relatively rare. In our practice, we see about one case in 1000 patients. The ratio of females to males is four to one.

ACUTE STRABISMUS FRANCESCHETTI TYPE[25,53]

This consists of a sudden onset of esotropia in adults without extraocular muscle paresis or significant refractive errors. Within a very short period, the angle may increase to large proportions.

Possibly, esophoria was preexistent. The stimulus for the sudden onset of esotropia may be psychic trauma or transient occlusion of the eye, which breaks up fusion. The eyes deviate into a convergent position of rest, producing bothersome diplopia. Since the double images are less bothersome the further apart they are, the angle of deviation increases (diplopia phobia of Van Der Hoeve).[64] As a result of this "flight from diplopia," the eyes overshoot the motor position of rest (escape strabismus of Mügge).[76] Such cases are not common in adults. Of 1102 esotropes, we know only two patients showing this picture. This type of strabismus occurs much more commonly in children after the second year of life. (See Essential Normosensorial Late Strabismus.)

VERTICAL DEVIATIONS

Vertical deviations are common with eso- and exotropia. The question arises whether these vertical deviations are primary, with a secondary horizontal deviation, or vice versa. The therapeutic approach depends upon which of these two events exists.

The question cannot be fully answered in many cases. Some types of strabismus do, however, provide points of orientation.

In severe oblique palsies, especially those that are congenital, there is commonly an expansion of the vertical fusional range if the deviation can be held latent, along with torticollis. The vertical deviation in these cases does not induce horizontal strabismus unless it is combined with a convergent position of rest or hypermetropia.

If there is significant loss of vision in one eye due to organic or traumatic damage, a horizontal deviation—either exotropia or esotropia—develops, ie, secondary strabismus. In these cases, one frequently sees a vertical component—specifically, elevation of the deviating eye. In some cases, after aphakia we have seen a consecutive "V" pattern with elevation in adduction. This indicates that the vertical acting muscles, either the recti or, more specifically, the obliques, are balanced by fusion, especially in their secondary positions. If fusion is lost, this imbalance of the vertical action becomes evident, especially in extreme positions of gaze, and vertical deviation develops.

If this vertical deviation is unilateral, then paralysis is the probable cause. If the vertical deviation is symmetric in both eyes, one is more likely dealing with dysfunction of the vertical muscles—for example, overaction of the inferior obliques. Three forms of vertical strabismus have to be differentiated from each other and from the general vertical deviations produced by paresis, alterations in the orbits, and other special types of vertical deviations.

ASSOCIATED OR CONCOMITANT VERTICAL DEVIATION

In associated or concomitant vertical deviation, the vertical deviation is the same in all directions of gaze. For example, one is dealing with right hypertropia that is 10 degrees in all directions. This rare form may be due to a difference in the vertical position of rest as a result of orbital or muscle tendon changes. Eye muscle paresis that has become fully comitant would be rare.

Dissociated vertical divergence—in other words, an elevation of the nonfixing or occluded eye—has been discussed under Congenital Strabismus. Oblique strabismus in the form of an elevation or depression of adduction has been described in the section on "A" and "V" patterns.

The last two types mentioned can be found in combination with each other. One should attempt to differentiate between the two components. Elevation on adduction (strabismus sursoadductorius) is muscular and due to overaction of the inferior oblique. It can be approached surgically. Dissociated vertical deviation is innervational, indicates very early onset of strabismus with poor binocular vision, and is less readily approached surgically. Of late, marked recession of the superior rectus of more than 10 mm (Jampolsky) or recession in combination with a posterior fixation suture (Knapp et al) has been advocated. Elevation of an eye is cosmetically more disturbing than depression of the same degree. This is due to the amount of sclera that is visible between the lower lid and the limbus on elevation which is not visible with depression. On the other hand, pseudoptosis can sometimes develop with hypotropia.

A particular type of vertical deviation can sometimes be seen with anisomyopia. The more myopic eye is depressed. This condition is known as "heavy eye," whereby the more myopic eye is "heavier" and therefore depressed.[8,138] The phenomenon of the heavy eye is rare. We have seen only one case in 1500 patients.

SPECIAL TYPES OF STRABISMUS

THE STILLING-TÜRK-DUANE RETRACTION SYNDROME[46,131,133]

The classic retraction syndrome consists of absent abduction and decreased adduction of the involved eye. Simultaneously, there is retraction of the globe into the orbit on adduction with narrowing of the lid fissures. In many cases, retraction is not very obvious, and the lack of abduction is the primary clinical finding.

This syndrome simulates abducens paresis. One should consider Duane's syndrome in all cases of abducens palsy in children.

Binocular function shows a characteristic behavior in most cases. Normal binocular vision with fusion is present in straight-ahead gaze and to the side of the uninvolved eye. Suppression develops on gazing in the direction of the paretic eye. This can be nicely demonstrated with the two-pencil pointing test. Children with this type of strabismus often have a head turn to allow single binocular vision. The head turn is in the direction of the underacting lateral rectus. In other words, in left Duane's syndrome, the face is turned to the left. Amblyopia is rare. The etiology of Duane's syndrome was formerly thought to be anatomic changes in the medial or lateral rectus muscle. In fact, at the time of surgery one frequently sees a positive forced-duction test with restriction of movement. Lately, electromyographic investigation has shown a disturbance of innervation in which the lateral rectus contracts simultaneously with the medial rectus (coinnervation). Recent investigations have shown that one is dealing with aplasia of the abducens nerve nucleus and that the lateral rectus muscle is innervated by branches from the oculomotor nerve.[68a] This explains the coinnervation. Formerly, one differentiated the convergent Duane type I from type II Duane's syndrome, in which the lack of adduction was most prominent. Considering the new information concerning lack of an abducens nucleus, it is simpler to accept either a convergent or a divergent starting position or position of rest for Duane's syndrome.[51] Cases have been described, however, for which a picture similar to Duane's syndrome developed after trauma or chemical burns. Therefore, a primary innervational disturbance cannot be assumed in every case.[101] The retraction syndrome can be combined with other syndromes, such as Klippel-Feil (fusion of cervical vertebrae) and the Goldenhar syndrome (preauricular tags, lid coloboma, epibulbar lipodermoids). These may be bilateral.

Surgery is indicated only if a marked esotropia or head turn exists. The operation of choice for convergent Duane's syndrome, in our opinion, is a small recession of the medial rectus combined with a small resection of the lateral rectus on the involved eye. With divergent Duane's syndrome, we perform a recession of one or both lateral recti. Besides this, there are a large variety of other surgical possibilities ranging from the Hummelsheim to the Faden operation. Each individual case has to be considered in relationship to its angle of deviation, restriction of movement, degree of retraction, and head position.

The incidence of Duane's syndrome in our practice is about one in 900 patients. Females outnumber males three to two. The left eye is more often involved than the right, in a ratio of nine to one.

DOUBLE ELEVATOR PALSY

The clinical picture consists of limitation of elevation of an eye. Both the superior rectus and the inferior oblique are underacting. Usually, the inferior oblique paresis is more obvious than the superior rectus underaction. In certain cases, Bell's phenomenon shows better elevation than voluntary upgaze. This indicates a supranuclear disturbance. We have been unable to find any obviously positive Bell's phenomena in our patients. Furthermore, we find it difficult to assume a supranuclear etiology for such a unilateral condition. One can differentiate three types of unilateral double-elevator palsy.

If single binocular vision is possible on downgaze, the chin is usually elevated and the head held back. Straight-ahead gaze and upgaze are avoided.

If fixation is done with the sound eye, the involved eye is hypotropic, and there is simultaneous ptosis—specifically, pseudoptosis of the upper lid on the involved side.

If fixation is done with the involved eye, the noninvolved eye is markedly hypertropic. Therapy consists of recession of the inferior rectus and resection of the superior rectus in the involved eye. True "double elevator" palsy patients almost always have pseudoptosis only. A ptosis operation may have to follow. Knapp and Dunlap recommend moving the insertion of the medial and lateral rectus in the involved eye up to the superior rectus.[48,78] Recession of the superior rectus on the uninvolved eye may also be considered.

THE BROWN SUPERIOR OBLIQUE TENDON

Brown's syndrome simulates paresis of the inferior oblique muscle. In adduction, the involved eye cannot rise above the midline. Sometimes it depresses spontaneously on adduction. Forced duction movement is also limited. One is dealing with changes in the tendon of the superior oblique muscle, which is too short or in which thickening prevents proper movement through the trochlea. With excessive tucking of the superior oblique tendon, iatrogenic Brown's syndrome occurs when the muscle body hits the trochlea.

In individual cases, difficulty in elevation may be only intermittently present. Sometimes on palpating the trochlea, one can feel a jerk as elevation occurs. There is an analogy in this symptom to "cracking" one's knuckles, which is also due to restriction of a tendon. A "click" phenomenon can occur.[123] These patients have parallel eyes and normal binocular vision on straight-ahead gaze and demonstrate problems only on upgaze. Others have partially accommodative esotropia with sensory changes.

Some cases of superior oblique tendon sheath syndrome have been described that spontaneously improved with time. We have had surgical success in patients for whom an operation was indicated by disinserting the superior oblique tendon.

PARETIC OR INCOMITANT STRABISMUS

In contrast to concomitant strabismus, paralytic strabismus is associated with restriction of mobility. While concomitant strabismus is primarily sensory or based on little-understood innervational disturbances, paralytic strabismus has a specific organic cause. This may lie in the orbit, in the sinus cavity, in the posterior cranial fossa, or supertentorially.

GAZE PALSY

Gaze palsy means limitation of simultaneous movement of both eyes. Since it involves both eyes, it rarely causes diplopia. The cause of gaze palsy is supranuclear. In horizontal gaze palsy, there is inability to move the eyes to the right or left. Total gaze palsy is usually present only with acute disturbances such as conjugate deviation occurring with stroke. Symptoms may range from total gaze palsy to isolated horizontal palsy manifest only by jerk nystagmus with a rapid component to the paralyzed side. The origin of the paresis is supranuclear, in either the region of the pons, the parapontine reticular formation, or the pathways from the frontal or occipital gaze centers of the brain to the pons.

Involvement of the frontal-lobe gaze center usually results in loss of voluntary movement. Occipital involvement causes loss of involuntary following movements. Diplopia is rare with horizontal gaze palsies.

With vertical gaze palsies, there is an inability of both eyes to look up or down. Upgaze is involved more often than downgaze. In more subtle cases, there is no limitation of vertical gaze but only a vertical jerk nystagmus with the rapid phase up. The location of the lesion is usually in the area of the mesencephalic reticular formation in the region of the oculomotor nerve. Vertical gaze palsies can be combined with disturbances in convergence and accommodation (Parinaud's syndrome). Since the vertical limitations may affect both eyes asymmetrically, diplopia is a common complaint in vertical gaze palsies that is not seen with horizontal gaze palsies.

Internuclear ophthalmoplegia is due to a unilateral or bilateral lesion in the posterior longitudinal fasciculus between the abducens nucleus and the contralateral oculomotor nucleus. For example, on left gaze, abduction of the left eye may be normal, but not adduction of the right eye. With convergence the medial rectus of the right eye works normally.

INFRANUCLEAR EYE MUSCLE PALSIES

Infranuclear eye muscle palsies can affect several muscles or only a single muscle. The lesion lies in the nerve to the muscle or in the muscle itself.

The etiology of eye muscle paresis in young patients includes trauma, infectious diseases, multiple sclerosis, and brain tumors. In older patients, the cause is usually a vascular disturbance such as hypertension, diabetes, or arteriosclerosis. The formerly very common syphilitic eye-muscle paresis has become rare. The degree of paralysis can vary markedly from total inaction to very subtle underactions of muscles that can only be appreciated in relationship to movements of the normal eye. The course of an eye muscle palsy varies. Nerves regenerate at the rate of one millimeter per day, and it may therefore take months for eye muscles to regain full function. In contrast to total recovery, paresis may be permanent or evolve into a concomitant strabismus.

One must keep Hering's law in mind in order to understand the events related to a muscle palsy. This law states that innervational impulses of similar degree go to the synergistic muscles of each eye. With a right superior oblique palsy, the nuclei send equally strong innervational impulses to that muscle as well as to the left superior oblique. The right superior oblique, however, because of defective conduction, receives less of an impulse. As a result, elevation of the right eye lags behind the left.

Weakness of the paralyzed muscle leads to overaction of its ipsilateral antagonist. For example, with palsy of the superior oblique on the right, overaction of the inferior oblique on the right develops. In time, this leads to secondary muscle contraction. Overaction of the contralateral synergist develops as well. In other words, with right superior rectus palsy, there is overaction of the left inferior rectus. This can lead to secondary paresis of its antagonist, the left superior rectus. These secondary deviations in eye muscle palsies are marked when the palsy has been present a long period of time and when the paretic eye fixes. If the nonparetic eye fixes, this usually leads only to contracture of the homolateral antagonist.

The angle of deviation is smaller when the nonparetic eye fixes than when the paretic eye fixes. One speaks of a primary angle of deviation when the uninvolved eye is used for fixation and a secondary angle when the paralyzed eye is used. The cause of these differences rests in Hering's law. It is important to remember that palsy of a muscle leads to contracture of the ipsilateral synergist and secondary inhibition of the contralateral antagonist.

The most important symptoms of extraocular muscle palsy are diplopia and compensatory ocular torticollis. The distance between the two images is greatest in the field of action of the involved muscle. The perceived second image is always in the direction opposite to that of the ocular deviation. For example, with right lateral rectus palsy, the right eye deviates nasally and the second image is localized temporally. When the right eye is elevated, the second image is depressed. If the right eye shows excyclotorsion — for example, with palsy of the right superior oblique muscle — the second image appears intorted. If paresis is not severe, the double images may be avoided by bypassing the field of action of the involved muscle. For example, with right lateral rectus palsy, right gaze is avoided. This leads to a head turn, specifically a right face turn. Subjectively, eye muscle palsies evoke strong complaints that may develop into dizziness and nausea. Occlusion of the involved eye brings immediate relief. On fixation with the paralyzed eye, there is often false localization of the object being fixated. The patient consistently points past the objects.

Of 166 ocular muscle palsies in our patient population, superior oblique palsy was the most common, at 44%. Lateral rectus palsy followed with 18%. This is in contrast to the majority of the literature, in which lateral rectus palsy is indicated as being most common. Superior rectus palsy occurred 7.8% of the time and the inferior oblique 7.2% of the time. (Admittedly, one-third of these were Brown's tendon sheath syndrome.) Medial rectus palsy occurred at a frequency of 4.8%; double elevator palsy of one eye, 4.8%; inferior rectus palsy, 3.6%; and oculomotor nerve palsy, 3%. In 6% of cases, the disturbance in mobility was due to maxillary fracture.

Abduction is compromised in lateral rectus palsies. The involved eye is adducted. Diplopia occurs with abduction. The second image is on abduction. The side of the paretic eye is therefore called "homonymous" or "uncrossed." The compensatory head position turns the face in the direction of the paralyzed muscle, turning the eye to the opposite side. With right lateral rectus muscle palsy, the face is turned to the right, eyes to the left. Abducens paresis can be bilateral.

With superior rectus palsy, paralysis of the elevator of the eye is most marked in abduction. For this reason, maximum diplopia in right superior rectus palsy appears on right gaze and upgaze. The compensatory head position consists of elevation of the chin, and face turned to the right. This leads to the position of the eyes being down and left. The involved eye is hypotropic.

Paresis of the medial rectus leads to restriction of adduction. The involved eye is abducted. Paresis of the right medial rectus causes maximum diplopia on left gaze. Diplopia is avoided by turning the face left, the eyes right.

Paralysis of the inferior rectus leads to the depression of the eye being marked in abduction. With right inferior rectus palsy, maximum diplopia is on right gaze and downgaze. The involved eye is hypertropic. To compensate, the eyes are turned left and up. This is achieved by depressing the chin and turning the face right. The involved eye is higher.

One must remember that the superior oblique has two primary functions, namely intorsion and depression. With paresis of the right superior oblique, maximum diplopia occurs when the right eye is depressed in adduction and with incyclorotation produced by tilting the head to the right shoulder. To avoid this position, the head is tilted to the left shoulder, the face is turned to the left, and the chin is depressed. This results in a gaze to the right and up. The involved eye is hypertropic. Superior oblique palsies can be bilateral.

With inferior oblique palsies, maximum diplopia occurs with the eyes in adduction and excyclorotation. For this reason, with right inferior oblique palsy, the head is tilted to the right shoulder, the chin is elevated, and the face is turned left, allowing right gaze and downgaze to avoid the double images. The involved eye is hypotropic.

In summary, there are four diagnostic clues: (1) elevation of the right or left eye, (2) increase in the vertical deviation on right gaze or left gaze, (3) increase on upgaze or downgaze, and (4) head tilt to the right or left shoulder. Each of these clues cut in half the number of muscles that could be at fault. With three steps, one can therefore arrive at the appropriate muscle. With hypertropia of the right eye, there is either paresis of a depressor of the right eye (superior oblique or inferior rectus) or paresis of an elevator of the left eye (inferior oblique or superior rectus).

If the vertical deviation increases on right gaze, one is dealing with palsy of either the right inferior rectus or the left inferior oblique. For the third step, one can choose — either increase vertical deviation on up- or downgaze, or use the head tilt test. With superior oblique palsy, it sometimes occurs that overaction of the inferior oblique is more obvious than underaction of the paretic superior rectus. In this case, deviation on elevation is greater than on depression, and for this reason it is best to choose the head tilt for the third step. If the right hypertropia is most marked on upgaze, the left inferior oblique is paretic. Right hypertropia greatest on right gaze and downgaze indicates palsy of the right inferior rectus. If the right hypertropia increases on left gaze, palsy of the right superior oblique or the left superior rectus is the cause. If the hypertropia is greatest on left gaze and downgaze, the right superior oblique is involved. If the right hypertropia is greatest on left gaze and upgaze, one must consider left superior rectus paresis. Similar considerations are true for the left eye.

Since paresis of the superior oblique leads to secondary palsy of the superior rectus of the other eye and vice versa, it is sometimes difficult to decide which muscle was affected first. The head tilt test of Bielschowsky helps to decide this.[65] On right head tilt, the intorters of the right eye are stimulated.

In determining the affected muscle that is the cause of diplopia, a variety of tests are useful, including coordinometry according to Hess, use of a binocular visual field, simple measurement of the ocular deviation and their excursions, recording of double images, and the three-step head tilt test. The two-pencil touch test allows one to determine quickly in which gaze of vision binocularity and stereopsis are present. Electromyographic investigations are interesting and elegant but require specialized laboratories. Their description as well as that of measuring saccadic velocities is beyond the scope of this book. In the case of a palsied superior oblique, this muscle is unable to carry out this intorsion, and its synergist for this action, the superior rectus, attempts to compensate, thereby overacting. This overaction of the right superior rectus leads to an increase in the elevation of the right eye. One tilts the head to the side of the suspected superior oblique and does an alternate cover test. If the vertical divergence has increased, this speaks in favor of superior oblique palsy.

A total third nerve palsy includes ptosis, and the position of the eye is down and out. There is marked restriction of the involved eye in the direction of adduction, elevation, and depression. Pupillary reaction is lost, and accommodation paralyzed. In many cases, only the extraocular muscles are paralyzed, with accommodation and pupillary reaction maintained. Ptosis is a sign of progressive peripheral nerve paralysis but appears last with progressive nuclear involvement. Innervation of the superior rectus muscle is crossed at the oculomotor nucleus. The levator of the lid is innervated bilaterally. The remaining muscles are innervated ipsilaterally. Total nuclear paralysis therefore involves the ipsilateral medial rectus, the inferior rectus, the inferior oblique, the pupillary sphincter and ciliary muscle, and the contralateral superior rectus. Ptosis does not develop because of the bilateral innervation.

External progressive ophthalmoplegia begins with bilateral ptosis followed by paresis of the extraocular muscles. This condition is rare. Isolated abducens or trochlear nerve paralysis by itself has no localizing value.

Unilateral underaction of the superior oblique and overaction of the inferior oblique can occur with plagiocephaly as a result of premature unilateral closure of the corona suture. The fontal eminence is missing on the involved side, and the orbit is displaced superiorly. Bilateral trochlear paresis is usually the result of trauma at the point of crossing of these nerves in the anterior medullary velum. Diplopia is not present on upgaze. Therefore, the patient assumes a typical chin-down position.

Bilateral abducens palsy is usually the result of increased intracranial pressure. Sometimes esotropia is obvious in this situation even though lack of abduction is not. One can speak of intracranial pressure esotropia. If multiple nerves associated with the extraocular muscles are affected, one is usually dealing with a problem in the carotid sinus or the superior orbital fissure.

The therapy for eye muscle palsies consists of medical as well as specific ophthalmologic treatment. Sensitive patients may be particularly burdened psychologically by eye muscle palsies, and empathy on the part of the physician is important. The patient's performance at his job or in tasks such as driving can be markedly reduced. The patients suffer all the more because those around them may have little understanding for their problem. The external signs are subtle, evoking less sympathy than obvious physical symptoms such as a limp. The patient must receive support and understanding from his eye doctor during this often-long period of healing. Even if therapeutic methods are of little value, they may have to be undertaken just for the psychic benefit of the patient.

General medical therapy should treat the underlying problem. This requires cooperation between ophthalmologist, neurologist, neurosurgeon, internist, and otolaryngologist.

Ophthalmic treatment is directed at eliminating diplopia. One should always attempt to maintain fusion in at least one position of gaze. This is sometimes possible by tilting the head. Many patients assume this head position unconsciously; others must be instructed to do so in order to learn in what head position they may see binocularly and singly.

If a head tilt is inadequate, then prisms are often useful. In prescribing prisms, one should avoid all dissociating tests. One should prescribe the minimal prism correction that allows binocular single vision in the primary position. Prisms may be incorporated into the glasses. Since the degree of prism correction varies markedly in the early course of muscle paresis, prescription of expensive ground in prisms and glasses should be avoided. One should use clip or paste-on prisms. For larger deviations, the segmented "Fresnel prisms" are useful in that they are thinner and lighter than normal prisms. They are commercially available in plastic as self-adhering Fresnel prism membranes.[74] Segmented prisms have the drawback of decreasing vision.

All prisms subjectively distort the patient's surroundings. This is particularly bothersome for walking, and patients must be alerted to it. Even if it is not possible to wear prisms full time, the patient should be instructed to wear them one to two hours per day in order to maintain binocular vision in a specific direction of gaze, thereby expanding this region. The prism correction should be checked regularly by the ophthalmologist.

Sometimes prescription of an opaque glass or occluder to eliminate diplopia cannot be avoided. One must remember that this disrupts fusional innervation, and that the fusional tone of the eye muscles and the tendency

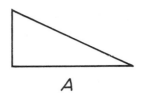

A

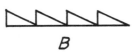

B

Fig. 67–
a) Regular prism; and
b) Fresnel prism.

Fresnel prisms are lighter and thinner. Particularly useful are the soft membrane Fresnel prisms made out of plastic. They can be pressed onto the glasses.

toward sensory cooperation are therefore ultimately lost.

Orthoptic exercises for expanding the fusional range can be used to support the home exercises. Active efforts to move the eyes in the direction of the paralyzed muscles are recommended. Unless one is dealing with a purely mechanical restriction, one must be careful with this, because overaction of the contralateral synergist will be strengthened just as much as the function of the affected muscle.

The majority of eye muscle palsies recover spontaneously. Surgery should therefore be avoided for at least six months after onset. In some cases, surgery cannot be avoided entirely. The surgery of choice is strengthening the paralyzed muscle, often combined with weakening its antagonist. In some cases, weakening the contralateral synergist is indicated. In the case of superior oblique palsy, for example, one could recess the contralateral inferior rectus. With total paralysis of the lateral rectus, a muscle transposition on the order of a Hummelsheim operation may be indicated.[72] This surgery consists of transferring one-third of the superior and inferior rectus to the lateral rectus.

Another surgical choice is the Jensen procedure. Here half the superior rectus and half the inferior rectus are joined with the appropriate halves of the lateral rectus via sutures.

EYE MUSCLE DISTURBANCES WITH ORBITAL INJURIES

Injuries of the facial bones and orbit can lead to disturbances in ocular motility with bothersome long-standing double vision. In the majority of cases, one is dealing not with a true palsy but with a "relative palsy." Such complications of ocular motor movement are becoming more and more common with the increase in head injuries due to traffic accidents. After severe accidental trauma, the generalized condition of the patient is initially critical—coma and cerebral contusion. Local fractures may be hidden by hematomas and edema. Traumatic strabismus is therefore often not apparent until weeks or months after an injury, when the patient is alert and well enough to complain of diplopia. The ophthalmologist is brought into the case at this point and must try to differentiate between various possibilities. These include orbital or muscle sheath hematomas caused by the trauma, leading to restriction of extraocular motility.

The so-called "blow-out fracture" results from blunt trauma elevating the intraorbital pressure, leading to a fracture in the weakest portion of the bony orbit, namely the floor. As this fracture occurs, the orbital contents, usually retrobulbar fat, are displaced into the maxillary sinus. The inferior rectus and inferior oblique may be trapped in the fracture of the orbital floor. Sensory examinations show skin hypoasthenia in the distribution of the infraorbital nerve. Enophthalmos and downward displacement of the involved eye are often combined with inability to elevate the eye.

A Le Fort's fracture involves the maxillary bone, the zygoma laterally, and the nasal bone medially. The facial bone structure on the involved side is displaced downward. The globe is also displaced inferiorly by several centimeters. A flattening of the cheek occurs.

The characteristic ophthalmic picture is that of limitation of elevation and sometimes a modest limitation of depression of the involved eye. The patient has diplopia on upgaze, but often is able to fuse on downgaze. For this reason, a head-back, chin-up position may be adopted for downgaze. Restriction can be greater on downgaze than on upgaze if the fracture is deep posteriorly in the orbit and the patient was looking up at the time of injury. Diplopia is greatest while reading, as opposed to other activities such as driving.

It is important that the fracture be repaired as rapidly as possible. This is usually done by the otolaryngologist or maxillofacial surgeon. If malocclusion of the teeth is present, oral surgery may be needed.

The situation may be very difficult when the fracture is old and diplopia still exists. Cooperation between ophthalmologist, maxillofacial surgeons, and otolaryngologist is needed. Ultimately, surgery on individual eye muscles may be indicated.

Prism glasses with base up on the involved side have proven very useful when surgery of the orbit and extraocular muscles has not led to full resolution of the problem. It is even possible to place prisms into bifocal glasses in such a way that their action is greater at distance than at near gaze. It is best to determine the number of needed prisms experimentally by first prescribing temporary paste or clip-on prisms.

MYOPATHIES

High Myopia Myopathy[71]

Not uncommonly, a marked limitation of extraocular movement develops in highly myopic patients, particularly women older than the age of 40.

Usually, one is dealing with a restriction of abduction that increases gradually. In extreme cases, this may develop to a point where both eyes are fixed in adduction. In order to fixate, the patient has to turn the head to such an extreme that glasses may get in the way of vision. The visual axis no longer passes through the glasses but is blocked by the nasal rim of the frames (strabismus fixus).

At the time of surgery, one discovers that passive abduction is restricted (positive forced duction) and may not improve much even after separating the medial rectus from the globe. Despite marked amounts of surgery, results are minimal. It is as if the globe were bound down in adduction through a posterior orbital staphyloma. It is not clear whether this is a true myopathy or only a relative weakness of the musculature related to the marked anatomic restrictions present. There is a relationship between the myopathy of severe myopia and the acute-onset strabismus of Bielschowsky. Certain cases begin as acute strabismus with diplopia at distance and then evolve into the clinical picture of myopathy.

The restriction in motility may be limited to one eye if unilateral myopia is present. Vertical deviations are common in this type of strabismus. If highly myopic anisometropia is present, the involved eye is usually hypotropic. In such cases, one speaks of a "heavy eye."[8,138] A myopathy of severe myopia was seen in our patient population in one out of 2000 patients. The average age of the patient was 49 years, and women outnumbered men in a ratio of 10 to 1.

Hyperthyroid Myopathy

Endocrine exophthalmos is often accompanied by difficulty in elevating the eyes. This may be bilateral and symmetric or may involve the more exophthalmic eye unilaterally. Vertical diplopia is common. The limitation of movement is specific for the superior rectus muscle. Histologic changes in this muscle have been described. One can also envision that the action of the superior rectus weakened by age is further compromised in a truly mechanical way by the exophthalmos.

In many cases, hypotropia of the eye and restricted upgaze are due purely to massive contraction of the inferior rectus. This muscle should then be recessed. It is crucial to remember that eye muscle paresis may precede any other clinical signs of hyperthyroidism. Computerized axial tomography and echography of the extraocular muscles allow one to differentiate between hyperthyroid- and neoplasm-induced changes.

Myositis

There are two types of myositis. Acute ocular myositis is accompanied by lid edema, exophthalmos, conjunctival hyperemia, chemosis, and pain. In contrast, chronic oligosymptomatic myositis appears as variable eye muscle palsies with diplopia and mild conjunctivitis. Its course is characterized by exacerbations and remissions.

Both these clinical pictures present a paradox in that marked restriction of movement occurs, while the electromyographic innervational patterns are normal. Therapy consists of local and systemic corticosteroids.

Pseudoparalytic Myasthenia Gravis

Myasthenia gravis usually presents as ptosis with superior rectus palsy. Complaints get worse late in the day, and are fewest in the morning. Rapid alternation of the ptosis from one eye to the other is pathognomonic. Symptoms of fatigue are typical: The upper lid droops on prolonged upgaze. The female/male ratio is three to two. Myasthenia may occur at any age but is most common in women in the third decade of life and in men in the sixth or seventh decade.

Myasthenia gravis is a disturbance of the conduction of impulses from nerve to muscle whereby acetylcholine is underactive. Anticholinesterases inhibit degradation of acetylcholine, normalizing nerve conduction. Therefore, Mestinon (pyridostigmine bromide) is used in the treatment of myasthenia. Proof of the diagnosis is the pharmacologic Tensilon (edrophonium chloride) test. Two milligrams of Tensilon are injected intravenously to test for an allergic reaction. If none occurs, two minutes later a total of 8 mm is injected. Electromyography done during this test gives objective confirmation of the diagnosis.

EXTRAOCULAR MUSCLE FIBROSIS

This is a congenital restriction of extraocular movements, which may be familial. The inferior recti are most commonly involved. The eyes are turned down, and the chin is tilted upward. Ptosis or pseudoptosis is present and may obscure the extraocular movement problem. To differentiate, one can elevate the upper lids with tape. If this fails to straighten the head, the diagnosis of fibrosis is confirmed.

On attempted upgaze, jerky convergent movements develop. Forced duction on elevating the globe is positive. Resection of the inferior rectus potentially with resection of the superior rectus and ptosis surgery is indicated. All extraocular muscles may be fibrosed, not only the inferior rectus.

EXTRAOCULAR MUSCLE MOTILITY DISTURBANCES WITH CRANIAL DYSOSTOSES

Plagiocephaly results from premature closure of the coronary suture resulting in hypertropia of the eye on the affected side. The clinical picture is one of a marked superior oblique palsy with overaction of the inferior oblique. The diagnosis is readily made because the frontal eminence is absent and the brow flattened. Overaction of both inferior obliques is common in Crouzon's disease.

OCULAR MOTOR APRAXIA
(COGAN, BALINT)

This is a disorder of horizontal eye movement. Patients are unable to make voluntary horizontal saccadic movements. The fixation reflex, however, is intact. In order to look at an object to his side, the patient must make head thrust movements in the direction of the object of interest. This overshoots the object but allows fixation of the object via reflex fixation. The affliction is most obvious when the child begins to sit up. It may disappear at approximately age five. Obviously, compensatory mechanisms develop at that time which mask the symptoms. The horizontal saccades in either direction are absent on optokinetic testing.

SUPERIOR OBLIQUE MYOKYMIA

This is a rhythmic spasm of the superior oblique muscle. It is most obvious on downgaze and inward gaze, appearing as a sudden vertical deviation with incyclorotation. The patient is bothered by the diplopia. The image of the affected eye is subjectively elevated and extorted. The cause is unknown. Treatment consists of Tegretol (carbamazepine). In one case, we had to excise the entire tendon of the superior oblique and weaken the ipsilateral inferior oblique muscle.

FIXATION LOSS, PHOTOPHOBIA, AND
STRABISMUS WITH CEREBRAL DAMAGE
AND SEVERE EPILEPSY[84]

Children with severe epilepsy and cerebral palsy (usually the result of perinatal asphyxia) demonstrate very obvious optomotor behavior. This is present even when antiepileptics are used. Gaze is almost never straight ahead but varies between downgaze, sidegaze, and upgaze. Correct fixation of an object does not take place. On fixation testing of the fundus, for example, with the star of an ophthalmoscope, the fixation object falls far in the retinal periphery and moves about. This is in contrast to immediate fixation of the object, which is done even by normal infants. The mothers are unable to maintain direct eye contact with the infants and say that the "eyes run away from the child." For this reason, these children are frequently considered to be blind. Their development is often retarded, and they demonstrate spastic changes. Later, as they are able to grasp objects, they do not fixate the object but make a sweeping eye movement across the object and then grasp it. As best tested, vision appears decreased.

Strabismus is common. It is usually esotropia but may sometimes be exotropia. Nystagmus may be present, but this is not obligatory. Optokinetic nystagmus cannot be obtained. The pupils react directly to light, and photic stimulation of the electroencephalogram is normal. Photophobia is common. The history helps in the diagnosis. Usually, a perinatal asphyxia led to cerebral damage with multifocal epilepsy. The patients are usually undergoing antiepileptic therapy, and questions concerning such medications need to be asked.

NYSTAGMUS

The word "nystagmus" is derived from the Greek *nystazein* which means "nodding." By nystagmus, one means a condition in which the eyes cannot be held still but have a constant tremulous movement.

A variety of mechanisms are needed to keep the eyes still. Since the eye is not fixed but is itself moveable within a moveable body, stabilization requires regulation through the vestibular system. In addition, the eyes need an optical point of fixation for the fovea. Proprioceptive end organs in the neck muscle and cerebellum exert tonic control on the ocular position. The cause of nystagmus can therefore be visual, within the labyrinthine system, or centrally, where these various influences are coordinated. Few symptoms in ophthalmology have such a multitude of potential causes as does nystagmus.

Certain characteristics are used to describe and evaluate the types of nystagmus. The movements may be regular, irregular, or chaotic. Their direction may be horizontal, vertical, or rotary. These directions may be combined in any variety of ways. The movements may have various frequencies and degrees of amplitude. With pendular nystagmus, the to and fro movements are equal. With jerk nystagmus, movement in one direction is more rapid than in another. Jerk nystagmus is classified according to the direction of the fast phase. For example, if both eyes slowly drift left with a subsequent rapid return to the right, one speaks of a right jerk nystagmus.

Normally, the eyes are not totally stationary while fixating on an object but have small invisible movements designed to avoid local adaptation. With congenital optical anomalies such as cataracts or organic macular hypoplasia with albinism, these normal fixation movements are accentuated and visible as nystagmus. This is referred to as amblyopic or ocular nystagmus.

The normal physiologic horizontal-jerk nystagmus present on extreme abduction is called "end point nystagmus." The rapid phase is in the direction of the object of regard (deviation of the eye).

Nystagmus can be induced by irritating the labyrinthine system. Sitting in the Bárány rotary chair, the subject has to tilt his head 30 degrees forward in order to place the horizontal labyrinth in a horizontal position. This labyrinth forms an angle of 30 degrees with the horizontal meridian posteriorly. During rotary movement, the eyes slowly turn opposite to the direction of rotation and return rapidly in a jerk fashion to the direction of rotation. With the person moving to the right in the chair, the endolymph flows left because of inertia.

On cessation of movement of the chair, endolymph continues to flow in the direction of prior chair movement, again because of inertia. This results in postrotary nystagmus with the slow phase in the direction of previous chair rotation and the return achieved in a jerklike fashion. Thus, the fast phase of nystagmus during rotation is in the same direction, and postrotation is in the opposite direction.

In infants, one can do vestibular rotatory nystagmus testing by holding the child at an angle 30 degrees to the horizontal, and then rotating him to the right or left while observing the horizontal nystagmus thereby elicited. In this way, it is possible to differentiate pseudoabducens paresis from true sixth nerve palsy.

One can also induce vestibular nystagmus with caloric testing. The subject must retroplace the head 60 degrees, which places the horizontal labyrinth vertically. The horizontal labyrinth borders the medial wall of the tympanic cavity. Caloric irrigation of the auditory canal with cold water cools the endolymph, which then sinks. Cooling of the right labyrinth canal slowly moves the eyes right, and there is a rapid refixation phase to the left. If one irrigates the right auditory canal with warm water, the lymph rises upward in the direction of the ampulla. This manifests as a rapid-phase nystagmus to the right.

The mnemonic COWS—Cold Opposite, Warm Same—is useful in remembering the normal results of caloric irrigation. Optical stimuli can also be used experimentally to produce nystagmus. Pendular nystagmus may be induced by visually following a pendulum or metronome. Historically, this optokinetic nystagmus was called "railroad nystagmus," whereby the eyes followed objects passing by and returned in a jerklike fashion in the direction of the train's movement. Use of a rotating drum (optokinetic drum) is an excellent way of inducing such a jerk nystagmus. The eyes slowly follow stripes or objects printed on the drum in the direction of the drum's movement and rapidly return in the opposite direction (fast phase).

Neurologic nystagmus usually has its seat in the brain stem or vestibular system. Vascular or inflammatory brain stem lesions such as neoplasms or demyelinating disease are the usual cause. Brain stem lesions usually begin less dramatically than vestibular lesions. However, the course is progressive and frequently causes increasing symptomatology, leading to diplopia. The hallmark of vestibular nystagmus is a rapid stormy onset and symptoms of dizziness that ultimately improve. Nystagmus also occurs with gaze palsies.

For example, with right gaze-palsy nystagmus, a rapid phase to the right is seen. Vertical nystagmus is characteristic of vertical gaze palsies.

Congenital nystagmus is usually pendular and develops at approximately the third month of life. The pendular characteristic may change with time into jerk nystagmus. The pendular movements are then obscured by fine fixation jerks. We have seen this transition repeatedly. Similarly, with decreased illumination at the slit lamp, we have observed that irregular fixation nystagmus has as its underlying cause a slow pendular nystagmus which increased to jerk nystagmus with normal illumination. One can assume that these fixation jerks develop on top of pendular nystagmus in the interest of better vision.

The visual prognosis depends upon the anatomic differentiation of the fovea. If it is well developed, the nystagmus may diminish, and ultimately good vision results. If macular hypoplasia is present, for example, with albinism, a poor visual result occurs. The question of macular differentiation is also important for binocularity. Patients with congenital pendular nystagmus but well-developed fovea have strabismus less commonly than those with nystagmus and albinism. Relatively good stereopsis can be demonstrated even with the random-dot test. If an albinotic fundus is present, strabismus is very common. It is worthwhile to investigate the fovea ophthalmoscopically and, if possible, to photograph it for documentation and inspection. Color vision should always be tested in these patients.

The amplitude of congenital nystagmus is not the same in all directions of gaze. Usually, there is a primary direction of gaze in which the eyes are most quiet. If this is not the straight-ahead position, then a compensatory head position is adopted to place the eyes in this optimal null point. For example, if the eyes are most quiet on right gaze of 50 degrees, the face is turned left that number of degrees to place the eyes in their best null point position. This head position can be improved by the prescription of prisms.

If the head turn is extreme, surgery (Kestenbaum's or Anderson's operation) is indicated. In this way, the null point position is shifted from gaze to either side to a more normal straight-ahead position. For example, if nystagmus is least with both eyes right, then one needs to move both eyes to the left. According to Anderson, one should recess the right lateral and left medial recti.[5] Kestenbaum recommends a resection of the right medial and left lateral rectus with recession of the left medial rectus and left lateral rectus.[76] The amount of surgery should be greater than that used for concomitant strabismus.

Characteristically, latent nystagmus is seen almost exclusively in association with strabismus. It is one of the hallmarks of the congenital strabismus syndrome. Its presence indicates that strabismus has been there since birth. When both eyes are open, the eyes are relatively quiet or have minimal nystagmus. Once one eye is occluded, however, nystagmus appears, with the rapid phase in the direction of the fixating eye. The amplitude is often greater with the amblyopic eye fixating. In very small children with fixation of the amblyopic eye, we have been able to observe very slow, almost spastic, adduction movement interrupted by a rapid phase of abduction back to straight-ahead gaze. Over time and with improvement of visual function, this nasal deviation becomes less obvious and slower. With time, the nystagmus may decrease in amplitude and frequency without disappearing entirely.

Latent Nystagmus

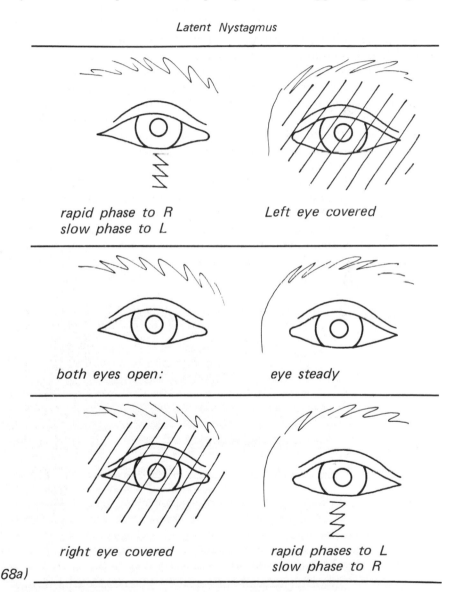

rapid phase to R
slow phase to L   Left eye covered

both eyes open: eye steady

right eye covered   rapid phases to L
                                   slow phase to R

68a)

Fig. 68–*a*) Latent nystagmus. 1. Left eye covered: rapid phase right, slow phase left; 2. Both eyes open, no nystagmus, right eye covered; and 3. Rabid phase left, slow phase right. *b*) Types of nystagmus. *c*) Torticollis and nystagmus corrected by prisms. *d*) Principle of the Kestenbaum procedure.

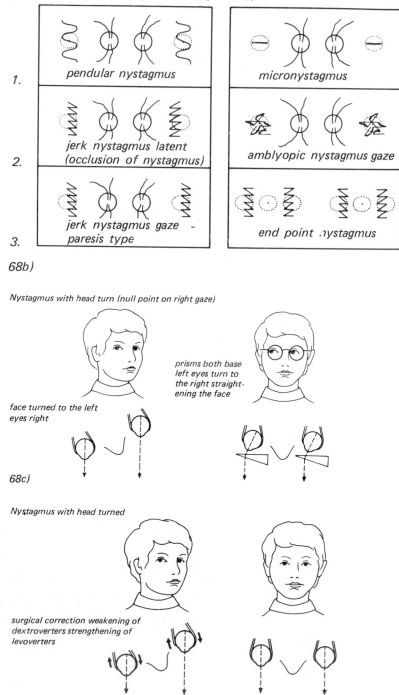

Nystagmus types

1. pendular nystagmus

2. jerk nystagmus latent (occlusion of nystagmus)

3. jerk nystagmus gaze - paresis type

4. micronystagmus

5. amblyopic nystagmus gaze

6. end point nystagmus

68b)

Nystagmus with head turn (null point on right gaze)

prisms both base left eyes turn to the right straightening the face

face turned to the left eyes right

68c)

Nystagmus with head turned

surgical correction weakening of dextroverters strengthening of levoverters

68d)

Latent nystagmus has to be looked for at the time of visual acuity testing. Visual acuity is markedly better with both eyes open than when one eye is covered. When one eye is covered, nystagmus develops or increases and visual acuity decreases. If one wishes to eliminate fixation on the part of one eye, one should not cover the eye but should use a strong "plus" lens that allows input of light but blurs vision. One has to be careful in the treatment of amblyopia if latent nystagmus is present. It is best not to use full-time patching but rather atropinization or graded occlusion of the fixing eye with glasses. If atropinization or partial occlusion is to work, full facial occlusion may be necessary.

The nystagmus blockage syndrome of Adelstein and Cüppers has to be included in the differential diagnosis of true and simulated abducens palsy in infants.[3] These authors claim that in 70% of the cases of convergence strabismus, nystagmus blockage is the origin of the strabismus. The hallmark of this syndrome is spontaneous nystagmus in the first months of life that decreases or disappears with the development of marked convergence strabismus. This convergence position may lead to secondary fibrotic changes and fixation of the globe in a position of adduction, giving the appearance of pseudoabducens palsy. The surgery recommended by these authors is retroequatorial myopexy (Faden operation).

Klipper differentiates the nystagmus blockage syndrome from "blocked nystagmus." With blocked nystagmus, one is dealing with variable angles of strabismus with head turns related to the nystagmus. The nystagmus sometimes is seen only at the extreme position of gaze, whereby end point nystagmus is superseded by fine jerk nystagmus. On placing a base-out prism in front of the fixing eye, the convergence angle of the other eye does not decrease. On horizontal gaze, the speed of movement is greater in the adducting eye.

We are most skeptical concerning this strabismus/nystagmus theory. Dampening of nystagmus by convergence is an old observation. That in rare cases this may lead to esotropia is undoubted. However, that 70% of esotropia should relate to this mechanism is unlikely. One also has to recognize that these authors have not differentiated between latent nystagmus and congenital pendular nystagmus. Latent nystagmus is associated with strabismus in 99% of cases and is one of the major symptoms of the congenital strabismus syndrome. Latent nystagmus is blocked not by convergence but by binocularity. With congenital pendular nystagmus, we have seen associate strabismus in only 30% of cases, and then usually without albinotic fundi. Fortunately, interest concerning the nystagmus blockage syndrome has lessened in recent years, and it appears as if it may ultimately be forgotten.

Monocular nystagmus may occur with amblyopia. We have seen unilateral vertical-jerk nystagmus with high degrees of myopia which improved after the amblyopia was corrected. In children with bilaterally decreased vision of unknown cause, a very fine vertical micronystagmus can frequently be observed ophthalmoscopically. This cannot be demonstrated on electronystagmography, and its nature is therefore largely unknown. An electroretino-gram should be done in these cases to rule out cone dystrophy.

4

THERAPY

GENERAL THERAPEUTIC GUIDELINES

Goal-oriented therapy can only be undertaken when the diagnosis is as specific as possible. Knowledge of various types of strabismus and their sensory changes is a prerequisite. Optimal therapy produces the best possible results with the least amount of effort. Treatment must be directed at restoration of binocular vision with minimum inconvenience to both parents and child.

Treatment of strabismus is not limited to a single therapeutic act. Instead, it is generalized long-term therapy, beginning with the first consultation and leading to the final permanent result. The time of treatment can last from the first few months of life to age 12 to 13.

Therapeutic measurements and their results are dependent not only upon the clinical aspect of the case but also on the overall personality of the child and the degree of compliance of the parents. The intelligence of the child, his willingness to undergo various therapeutic measures, and his active cooperation are major factors. Equally important is any underlying medical condition that may take therapeutic precedence, for example cerebral palsy, or that may prevent intensive orthoptic therapy such as epilepsy or disposition migraine.

The attitude of the parents is crucial. Occlusion therapy is carried out by the mother and not by the doctor. The child will not wish to wear glasses if the parents themselves are against the idea of glasses. Not all parents are able to carry the cost financially (prism glasses, bifocal glasses, hospitalization, and orthoptic training) or time expenditures equally.

The overall social and familial situation as well as the mobility of the population in this day and age, in which treatment is interrupted by changes in location and therefore in the doctor, also plays a role. After the first or second visit, the physician should have a clear idea of immediate and long-term goals as well as the treatment required to reach them.

The entire course of treatment can be subdivided into three stages, with appropriate intermediate goals.

Treatment of amblyopia should lead to good vision in each eye. Alignment of the eyes with either glasses or surgery has a cosmetic goal and is a prerequisite for the development of normal binocular vision.

Binocular cooperation should be achieved either on the basis of obtaining a small angle with anomalous retinal correspondence or on attaining true parallelism with normal binocular vision. The term "normal binocular vision" implies true complete parallelism of both eyes. This is in contrast to the term "binocular single vision," which can occur both in normal eyes and with abnormal retinal correspondence.

In adults, ocular motility problems are usually of different origin than in children. Frequently, one is dealing with a purely cosmetic reason for the surgery. Another important area is treatment of ocular muscle palsies, which can lead to severe restrictions of work capacity due to bothersome diplopia. A further group of patients consists of those who have severe headaches because of heterophoria or convergence insufficiency.

The physician not only needs to have the necessary knowledge for the treatment of these patients but also has to have the time required to carry out the therapeutic plan. Although a great portion of the treatment can be carried out by the parents at home, it is useful for the ophthalmologist to have an orthoptist available who has the time and patience to perform vision and binocular testing in children and to explain to the parents the rationale of individual treatments.

PRESCRIPTION OF GLASSES AND MIOTICS

Glasses are a burden for both parents and child. Nonetheless, for most children with esotropia, glasses cannot be avoided. One should prepare both parents and the child for the ultimate wearing of glasses. It is important to break down parental resistance to glasses and to alleviate their fear of injury. Ocular injury from wearing of glasses is rare. Often, the glasses act as a guard against injury. The split-second that an object is delayed by striking the frame is sometimes enough to prevent eye injury. Glasses injury is more common to the lid, nose, or eyebrows. For safety reasons, plastic lenses are preferred by most parents. They do have the drawback of being less scratch-resistant than glass lenses, however. We have had success in prescribing tinted or phototropic lenses for children who are very photophobic. Phototropic lenses do have an increased risk of shattering.

A major problem is the availability of adequately fitting frames for small infants. Because of the lack of development of a nasal bridge in infants and small children, the glasses are constantly slipping down the nose and need frequent refittings by the optician. An elastic strap such as an athletic strap is useful. Glasses should be fitted so that they extend well above the eyebrows of the child. In this way, small patients, who have to look up more than adults, are not tempted to look over their glasses.

To acclimate small children to glasses, it may be useful to start with sunglasses, especially during atropinization. If the child likes the sunglasses, he will also wear the corrective glasses, especially if the parents are enthusiastic about the "child's pretty glasses." It is helpful especially with hyperopes to give atropine at the time of dispensing the glasses. Even small children are aware at that point that wearing the glasses provides better vision. The earliest time period for wearing glasses is highly variable. Very small children with severe myopia will wear glasses gratefully. Severe hyperopes also accept the glasses well if one atropinizes them at the same time. Cerebrally damaged children, especially those unable to keep their head upright, will have difficulty in wearing glasses. The wearing of glasses is problematic as long as the child is not walking but crawling. The wearing of glasses is equally difficult during gymnastics, skiing, and swimming, and at summer camp. Lack of tanning around the eyes is proof that children are or are not wearing their glasses.

It is a general rule that hyperopia and astigmatism should be fully corrected for esotropes. This rule is primarily true for accommodative strabismus. A decrease of the retinoscopic value by half a diopter is allowable. Atropinized retinoscopy should be repeated annually. A common regimen is 0.5% atropine drops used three times daily for three consecutive days. Retinoscopy values are difficult to obtain in small children and are therefore somewhat inexact. From year to year, this improves, and new glasses should then be prescribed.

A certain degree of common sense has to be used with the prescription and wearing of glasses. Not all strabismic children need glasses, but when they are indicated, they must be insisted upon firmly with follow-ups to insure compliance.

Congenital strabismus occurs within the first year of life and is usually nonaccommodative. At this time period, therefore, glasses are not visually indicated but still may be needed. At one and one-half years of age, however, newly developing strabismus often has a marked accommodative component. Similarly, preexisting strabismus may develop an acquired accommodative angle at this time. Prescription of the full hyperopic correction at this age is therefore necessary.

A common misconception is that hyperopia is most marked at birth and decreases year by year thereafter. An ophthalmologist holding this viewpoint may therefore tell the parents that the glasses can be weakened over the years. We have made an opposite observation, however, and agree with others (Slapater, Brown, Andrée) that hyperopia increases up to the eighth year of life.[6,21,29] In any case, it is useful to tell the parents that one will probably have to increase the strength of the glasses over time. Decrease in the glasses' strength can be expected only after age 12. If not warned in this way, the parents may misinterpret the increase in strength of the glasses as a worsening of the child's condition and lack of progress.

One can deviate from the principle of full correction in those cases in which the strabismus is intermittent. In children older than age four, the correction can be as weak as possible, just strong enough so that the eyes remain straight. With younger children, hyperopia has to be fully corrected, however. The complaint of parents that their child only squinted intermittently prior to the prescription of glasses but did so constantly and to a greater degree thereafter must be anticipated. Prior to this, the child avoided accommodation to avoid diplopia, preferring blurred vision to double vision. After glasses, the child rejects the blurred vision existing without the glasses and accommodates more, inducing the turning. It is a pseudoworsening of the problem, about

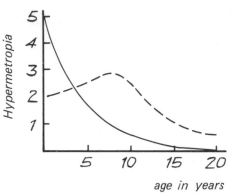

Fig. 69–Development of refraction in a child.
1. Solid line: after Chavase; and
2. Dotted line: actual course.

which parents must be forewarned. One must also explain to the parents that accommodative strabismus has a tendency to get worse over the first ten years of life.

True orthotropia with full correction is not common. Only 5% of our patients with esotropia were fully accommodative.[90]

Attempts to eliminate the residual angle by use of prisms in partially accommodative esotropia have failed in our experience. The residual angle is maintained by anomalous retinal correspondence. In those children whose eyes are straight for distance but continue to be esotropic at near gaze, bifocals are indicated. The bifocal segment must be set considerably higher than in adults. The bifocal line should bisect the pupil. Bifocal glasses are well tolerated by children. The near correction is usually +2.50 diopters but can be less when the weaker bifocal allows parallelism at near gaze. Attempts to reduce the bifocal strength over a period of time should be made in order to stimulate accommodation.[23,77] In patients with fully accommodative esotropia, one should attempt to teach relaxation of accommodation. In this way, the patients can become somewhat independent of the glasses. This is useful in certain situations, for example, at the swimming pool or in the bedroom. Naturally, without glasses, their vision is blurred, but their eyes do not cross.

Cases of severe hyperopia without esophoria or exotropia should not be fully corrected. Bilateral amblyopia secondary to astigmatism requires full astigmatic correction. Children with severe degrees of anisometropia will tolerate the full correction very well.

Contact lenses are indicated in unilateral childhood aphakia. Especially with traumatic cataracts, one should minimize the time between surgery and prescription of the contact lenses. Otherwise, the aphakic eye will rapidly become amblyopic, developing exophoria and cyclophoric tendencies. This disrupts the coupling of accommodation and convergence. If one waits months or years, fusion and parallel eyes may no longer be achievable, even with contact lenses and strabismus surgery. With axial anisometropia and anisomyopia, contact lenses are only rarely indicated. Theoretically, glasses in this situation provide less aniseikonia, since they are at the anterior nodal point. Contact lenses have the advantage of eliminating prismatic aberration on side gaze. Children tolerate aniseikonia very well.

Glasses are indicated in the first years of life with bilateral congenital severe myopia. A full correction should be achieved for exotropes with astigmatism, anisometropia, or myopia. If hyperopia in exotropia is present, its correction with "plus" lenses increases the tendency toward divergence. In certain cases, overcorrection with "minus" glasses is indicated to decrease the deviation.

Some years ago, miotics rather than hyperopic glasses were recommended for esotropia. These range from weak pilocarpine to stronger anticholinesterases such as Phospholine Iodide (echothiophate iodide). At times, this therapy is continued for years.[1,70] We do not agree with this. Short periods of treatment with miotics may be indicated postoperatively or as a compromise during swimming season or ski vacations. Long-term therapy, however, is rarely indicated, since full parallelism of the eyes is not achievable solely with miotics. Moore found full parallelism achievable with use of DFP drops in only 3.7%.[104]

Small angles are notorious for not alternating, and the danger of amblyopia is therefore great if total parallelism is not achieved. In that case, glasses and alternate patching are indicated. Furthermore, the danger of strong miotics must be recognized. Pupillary cysts can develop even in the face of concomitant Neosynephrine (phenylephrine hydrochloride) use. When these are seen, stopping the medication is indicated, and most cysts will regress. Lens opacities allegedly do not develop in children, but observation over decades may provide a different viewpoint of this question as well. It seems more appropriate to us to educate both parents and child in the wearing of glasses whenever possible rather than use miotics.

AMBLYOPIA TREATMENT

Treatment of amblyopia is one of the most important and satisfying therapeutic procedures an ophthalmologist can carry out. The earlier squinting children are diagnosed, the easier and more successful the therapy. After six months of age, it should no longer happen that children are not immediately brought to an ophthalmologist if they still squint. Reassurance that the strabismus will spontaneously improve or is not treatable until the third year of life is no longer acceptable. It should never occur that an ophthalmologist dismisses a strabismic child without diagnosis or treatment because "he is too young to do anything." In the case of alternating strabismus, one can wait and observe. However, in unilateral strabismus, one has to intervene. If one is not in a position to evaluate or treat small children, they should be referred to an interested colleague. A number of children will be referred to an ophthalmologist for pseudostrabismus. Both the referring physician and the parents should be congratulated for the appropriateness of the visit in such cases. If no clear diagnosis can be made, one should see the patient again in a few months. Under no circumstances should one undertake any therapy in pseudostrabismus, even if the parents insist.

When possible, amblyopia should be detected before school age. We have repeatedly observed how difficult proper amblyopia treatment is while the child is going to school. It is nonetheless indicated. It has to be pointed out to parents, children, and teachers that poor school performance because of the patching is transient and can be overcome later, while the amblyopia cannot. On the other hand, one needs to know the limits of amblyopia therapy and not unnecessarily undertake hopeless treatment.

Diagnosis of amblyopia can be made easily when an obvious strabismus exists. In order to detect amblyopia ex anisometropia and microstrabismic amblyopia, all young children should have vision testing as early as possible. This is usually practical at age three, and in the elementary school years. Since these amblyopic types are often familial, siblings of strabismic children should be seen immediately. The Lang stereo test is useful in detecting strabismus and amblyopia in such young children. Patients with amblyopia ex anisometropia frequently perform well on the stereo test compared with patients with microtropia.

A whole variety of amblyopia treatment methods exist, ranging from simple atropinization to active treatment with optical instruments. It is self evident that these are best applied in a stepwise fashion beginning with the simplest methods least bothersome to patients and parents. Success is dependent not only upon the treatment method used but also upon the depth of the amblyopia and its resistance to therapy. Resistance to therapy can vary greatly among different types of amblyopia. The earlier the onset and the longer the delay before therapy is begun, the more resistant to treatment is the amblyopia. Treatment is even more difficult when anisometropia or a motor anomaly is present. The course of improvement varies greatly. On the one hand, there are those small children who with very short periods of patching develop deep amblyopia and loss of central fixation in the patched and formerly dominant eye. On the other hand, there are individuals who even after months of patching immediately go back to fixing with the patched eye once the patch is removed. They may never achieve free alternation.

Full-time patching, ie, full-time occlusion with an adhesive skin patch, is the principal form of treatment. Patching is as essential to treating amblyopia as water is to fighting fires. The success of patching is directly related to the degree of compliance on the parts of parents and child.

Patching requires either the complete elimination or weakening of visual impulses to one eye. This may be achieved in various ways. With skin patching, one eye is directly covered by an adhesive bandage. Commercial patches for this purpose are available. Facial patches can be worn a number of days and nights until they begin to loosen themselves. It is unnecessary to remove the patch every evening at bedtime. A fair amount of time will be lost the next day in reapplying the patch. Furthermore, with frequent removal of the patch, the skin becomes irritated.

Facial patching is particularly indicated for deep amblyopia in the child who will immediately attempt to remove any glasses with occluders or in small infants not yet able to wear glasses. It is helpful to hold both the child's hands immediately after the occlusion is put on so that he does not immediately rip off the patch. The child should then be distracted by playing games or taking a walk. Occasionally, it is necessary to use arm restraints similar to those used with eczema to prevent scratching. Closure of the lids with Cyanacryl adhesives has been advocated.

With patching, psychologic support of the parents by the ophthalmologist and orthoptist is important via appropriate follow-up. For this reason, we almost never prescribe patches primarily but begin with atropinization of the good eye for about one month. We explain to the parents that if this does not lead to alternation, then on the next visit full-time facial patching would be recommended. If alternation fails to occur, the parents are psychologically prepared for the facial patching. Not infrequently, atropinization will lead to alternate fixation whereby the formerly amblyopic eye fixes at near gaze and the atropinized eye at distance. If this is the case, then one can continue with atropinization. After a period of time, we reduce atropinization. At first atropine is used daily, then every second day, and finally every third day. Ultimately, alternating atropinization (for example, Mondays and Tuesdays of the first week in the right eye and then in the opposite eye on the same days of the following week) is introduced. Such an alternating rhythm has to be coordinated with the duration of the atropinizing effect. This treatment is carried out until the child alternates spontaneously even without the atropine. The earlier the onset, the greater the chance that child is able to alternate spontaneously without atropine. Sunglasses can be worn, since small children are usually very photophobic during such treatment. If a small child readily wears sunglasses in this way, it is an indication that corrective glasses would also be tolerated.

If after several weeks of atropinization a shift in fixation does not develop, then patching therapy must be begun. If the child wears glasses, occlusion of the glasses may be attempted first. With deep amblyopia, however, the child will take off the glasses and will look over or around them even with the good eye atropinized. Usually, in such cases one starts out with full-time facial patching. If this is tolerated over a period of days, one can then go back to occlusion with glasses and atropinization.

Occlusion with glasses is less difficult for the parents than facial occlusion. One can use it only when visual acuity has improved to a certain point, since the child with deep amblyopia will look around the glasses. It is useful to atropinize the dominant eye in this transition between skin patching and occlusion with glasses. Other methods such as use of pirate patches or plastic occluders that fit on the back side of glasses may be useful. Placing an adhesive patch directly on the glasses or using paper or plastic tape on the lenses is often adequate.

With total occlusion, visual impressions reaching the eye are totally eliminated, as with facial patching. The central visual area can also be blocked, as with nontransparent occlusion placed on the glasses. Total occlusion is often not necessary; simply decreasing the quality of the image, called "partial occlusion," is useful. One can achieve this most easily with atropinization. Naturally, this works better with hyperopia or emmetropia than with myopia. For partial occlusion on glasses, one can use clear fingernail polish or semitransparent paper tape. Specifically designed for this is the occlusion material of Bangerter.[10] These are plastic sheets that paste onto the back of the lens. The transparency of these sheets is graded in eight steps from 20/200 to 20/20. One therefore applies them according to the depth of amblyopia.

Graded occlusion can be undertaken by gradually increasing the density of the filters (sneaking up), or vice versa, by gradually reducing filter density (sneaking out).

Constant occlusion is usually worn over long periods of time. There are cases, however, for which part-time occlusion is indicated, for example, one-half hour per day. That half-hour is usually best coordinated with visual tasks such as tracing, coloring, watching television, or playing video games.

Alternate fixation is the rule for congenital or early-infancy onset strabismus. Amblyopia tends to develop at a later time. We have observed many children who at first alternated but then at approximately one year of age became monocular strabismics with subsequent amblyopia. We therefore make it a rule to follow strabismic infants carefully, usually every three months. The parents are instructed to look for spontaneous alternation.

Since amblyopia is suspected with unilateral strabismus in a small child, one should attempt to convert monocular strabismus into alternating strabismus. This goal is reached when the child alternates freely. The simplest method with which we begin is to teach the mother to cover the fixing eye of the small child with her hand while he is drinking from a bottle.

Even after long periods of direct facial occlusion, there are infants who still fixate eccentrically with the amblyopic eye. This is often accompanied by inadequate or no abduction movement. In these cases, one should not wait but should surgically straighten the eye fixed in adduction. Amblyopia therapy has to be continued afterward.

Most authors agree that patching of the preferred eye should be carried out in infants and children up to three years of age regardless of the fixation pattern. There is equal unanimity concerning the need to patch the good eye of a child in the face of central fixation with an amblyopic eye at any age. Such an "unite de doctrine" is not present for the treatment of eccentric fixation after the third year of life.

Cüppers and Bangerter have recommended inverse occlusion; that is, occlusion of the amblyopic eye until active amblyopia treatment with optical devices is possible. They believe that if one occludes the dominant eye, eccentric fixation may become deeply seated in the amblyopic eye. This could worsen the prognosis for subsequent active amblyopia treatment. Nowadays, most authors recommend full-time occlusion of the fixing eye up to school age on the premise that such occlusion gives better results than the later use of active instrumentation for amblyopia (pleoptics).

If central fixation has not developed after several weeks of occlusion (increasing up to one-half hour per day), the occlusion therapy should be stopped. Intensive pleoptic therapy, for example, with a Euthyscope or Pleoptophor, may be considered.

What further treatment should be attempted after amblyopia with eccentric fixation has been cured? Conventional wisdom has it that one should try to establish normal binocular vision with perfectly straight eyes. In this way, it is guaranteed that visual acuity in the amblyopic eye is not lost.

Treatment to reach such a goal is lengthy and bothersome to the patients. Alternate occlusion over a period of a year is required to avoid development of anomalous retinal correspondence. Furthermore, surgery or prisms are needed to align the visual axis, with subsequent visual training on a binocular instrument. It has been our experience that we are unable to achieve this goal with these methods, and we therefore prefer to use alternate therapy.

Once optimal visual acuity is attained in each eye, occlusion is not suddenly interrupted. Children will frequently complain of diplopia if this occurs. This calls for recurrence of suppression and amblyopia. One should therefore try to achieve alternation.

Our method of choice for this is progressive decreasing occlusion with variable density occluders (sneaking-out occlusion).[10] This sneaking-out occlusion can be carried out unilaterally or alternately. For example, if the amblyopic eye has reached an acuity of one and this vision has been maintained with daily alternating occlusion, we then begin to decrease occlusion using a partial optic occlusion filter density of 0.1 (20/200). For a number of months, we occlude on a daily ratio of one to one and then eventually three to one. For a few additional months, we will use an occluder of 0.3 (20/70) visual acuity density. Finally, in the early school years, we stop using occluders, allowing vision of 20/20.

This graded optical occlusion is continued until the child is able to read fluently with either eye. Usually, this is the case by ten years of age. On discontinuing occlusion, the patient has to be rechecked after a few months to be certain that visual acuity remains stable. This type of graded occlusion has the advantage that one can carry it out over a period of months or years, during which the parents have proof that progress is being made as the density of the occluders is decreased.

We have repeatedly seen individuals who had a visual acuity of 20/20 in the formerly amblyopic eye who still have great difficulty reading with that eye. They read haltingly and complain that the text is unclear and moves about. We call this "reading amblyopia," since amblyopia is not detected with optotype testing but only on reading text. Reading is an important goal of our amblyopia therapy. It is therefore important to reach true alternation in the first few school years through use of alternating occlusion, thereby forcing the child to read with either eye. With good visual acuity in each eye, an occluder of optical density still allowing 20/20 vision is adequate and has the advantage that it is virtually invisible on the glasses. When alternation is achieved using a 20/20 occluder, this indicates that amblyopia is truly cured. At the same time, harmonious anomalous retinal correspondence with a small angle is allowed to develop.

Exercises employing red/green glasses are also useful in learning alternation.

Often, occlusion for a limited period of time each day is prescribed—for example, an hour a day while watching television or reading. A useful exercise is to check off all the "E's" in a text being read. This provides control of compliance, since the work can be checked on a return visit. It is useful to begin with large type and then go to progressively smaller type.

An additional home exercise consists of tracing with a red pencil. A red filter is worn in front of the better eye during this exercise. In this way, the red color can be seen only by the amblyopic eye.

In our experience, we have repeatedly seen that exercises and time-limited occlusion are done for only short periods of time. There is lack of compliance, particularly when no visible progress is being made. Pseudoabducens palsy generally cures itself spontaneously. Generally, graded optical occlusion is more acceptable and practical. Graded optical occlusion has also proven useful in amblyopia ex anisometropia. The danger of occlusion strabismus developing is less with graded occlusion than with total patch occlusion. We see little use for partial alternate occlusion in infants who spontaneously alternate as an effort to improve abduction in cases of pseudoabducens palsy.

Amblyopia treatment is not limited to the methods described here. A large number of others have been reported. For example, occlusion of the good eye combined with use of inverse prisms worn in front of the amblyopic eye, as recommended by Pigassou, with the prism base out on the amblyopic eye (after Cüppers), and prisms base-out on the amblyopic eye with patching of the good eye (Rubin).[39,116] Deller combines penalization with prisms base-out in front of the fixing eye.[42] It has also been recommended to place a red filter in front of the amblyopic eye while patching the good eye. This is to stimulate the red-sensitive color cones in the macula.[18] Atropinization of the good eye is supposed to be more effective with concomitant miotic usage of the amblyopic eye. Finally, in special cases of eccentric fixation, surgery has been recommended.[36,128]

Recently, penalization methods have been reported and emphasized. This is based on an observation of Pfandl, who noticed a near-distance alternation with normal retinal correspondence in some anisometropic children.[114] Artificial anisometropia is produced in the hope of stimulating near-distance alternation. With so-called "near penalization," the fixing eye is atropinized while the amblyopic eye is overcorrected by +3.00 diopters. It has been shown, however, that with high degrees of amblyopia, this method is inadequate to produce distance and near alternation. Patching therapy has to precede penalization in these cases. Penalization can then be used for the final stages of visual improvement and to reinforce the achievement of patching.[119],[120]

With distance penalization, "plus" lenses are placed in front of the fixing eye to blur objects at a distance. Besides these two basic methods, there are a whole series of modifications that vary from author to author. The advantage of penalization is that children who normally would resist wearing their glasses wear them willingly because of the atropinization. This can also be achieved simply with atropinization of the good eye. In our experience, "plus" lenses for near vision are not mandatory. A criticism of penalization would be that it hinders accommodation. This may be desirable in cases of extreme convergence excess.

Additionally, marked hypermctropia (the origin of which is unclear) has bcen observed to occur with long-term atropinization and simultaneous blocking of accommodation. This prolonged cycloplegic treatment prevents

Fig. 70-Graded occlusion.

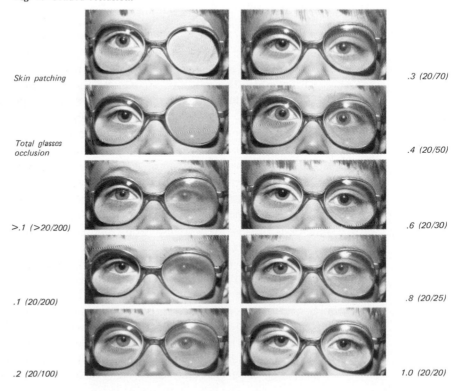

Skin patching

Total glasses occlusion

>.1 (>20/200)

.1 (20/200)

.2 (20/100)

.3 (20/70)

.4 (20/50)

.6 (20/30)

.8 (20/25)

1.0 (20/20)

the natural ametropization process. Thus, the great results one hoped to achieve with penalization have not occurred. Normalization of abnormal retinal correspondence is not achievable by the penalization method. For this reason, we almost always prefer graded occlusion to penalization. It is not necessary to replace the venerable and clear term atropinization with the modern term penalization. For some time, it has been popular (especially in France, under the influence of Berrondo) to use sectorial and variously shaped occluders placed upon glasses. This relates back to the ancient binasal sectoral occlusion and represents a complicated adaptation of this to attempt to achieve alternation and treatment of complicated muscular overactions. Forty different possibilities of overacting patterns are recommended, which automatically condemns this method.

Instrumentation amblyopia therapy, such as pleoptics, is beyond the capacity of the average ophthalmologist. It is optimal to have the child undergo three therapy sessions a day for approximately three weeks. The treatment triad of Bangerter is Pleoptophor, localizer, and zentrophor, or the afterimage treatment of Cüppers with a Visuscope in combination with the coordinator.[11,34,130] Since prognostically favorable cases react well to occlusion therapy, instrumentation is usually reserved for difficult cases with a poor prognosis. This should be remembered in assessing results. Results of all these techniques have been disappointing, including those of the CAM trainer. The rule for amblyopia therapy should be: Achieve optimal function with minimal effort!

SURGICAL TREATMENT

Eye muscle surgery has been tremendously popular since 1839, when Johann Friedrich Dieffenbach first did a myotomy of a medial rectus muscle without general or local anesthesia. Strabismus surgery still has a number of unsolved problems and variables, however. It is impossible to describe more than a few key concepts. Generalizations in the area of surgery are dangerous, and no magic formula can replace careful analysis of individual cases and the intelligent application of the surgeon's experience.

First of all, one has to define the goal of surgery in early cases. If normal binocular vision is to be achieved, the eyes must be made parallel. If there is no hope for normal binocular vision and the sensory goal is functional binocularity on the basis of abnormal retinal correspondence, then the surgical goal is to create a small residual angle of deviation. If there is no hope for anomalous binocular vision, then a cosmetically acceptable angle is the aim. Here, too, one usually attempts to achieve a small residual esotropia.

The time indications for performing surgery are variable. In cases of normosensorial, late-onset, infantile late strabismus and with severe cosmetic deformities, the need for surgery is more pressing. In other situations, it is better to defer surgery until after many examinations and a long period of observation. One must remember that with time there can be a spontaneous improvement in esotropia as the position of rest of the eyes in the skull becomes divergent with growth.

The timing of strabismus surgery revolves primarily around the question of whether surgery should be performed early or at an age when orthoptic treatment is feasible. There are authors who would operate immediately, ie, after six months of age, since this leads to the best binocular visual results.[30] We do not agree with this viewpoint, since we have seen poor results in congenital squint syndrome cases. The angle of deviation is often not constant in these children in the first two years of life but changes, with later divergence or increased convergence. Additionally, there is the danger that a high-grade strabismic amblyopia may develop, since the parents see what cosmetically appear to be orthotropic eyes. They think that a full cure has been achieved and do not keep follow-up appointments. An alternate recommendation is to defer surgery until four to six years of age because of the belief that only at this age one can achieve an exact diagnosis. Proper orthoptic or pleoptic therapy can often be carried out. This viewpoint requires the eyes to be totally occluded on an alternating basis up to the time of surgery in order to prevent anomalous retinal correspondence. In our experience, this is an error, since it is too much to disrupt normal binocular vision in its developmental period and then expect it to function normally at a later date.

The older viewpoint, that one should wait until age ten or twelve for strabismus surgery, is outdated. In cases in which surgery is for cosmetic reasons only and spontaneous exotropia can be expected (ie, unilateral amblyopia), it may be wise to defer surgery as long as possible.

In those rare patients in whom amblyopia that resists patching may be present, it is best to operate early. In these cases, the eccentrically fixing eye is more-or-less held in adduction and remains in this position even after occlusion of the leading eye. For this, we recommend surgery on the amblyopic eye within the first year of life. Patching of the good eye is begun immediately after surgery. One can safely wait in cases of alternating congenital strabismus.

Parents are often bothered by large angles of deviation. This is reinforced by comments from others. In this case, one should operate at about two and one-half years of age. Cosmetically bothersome deviation should certainly be eliminated before the child is aware of his deformity and suffers due to the comments and attitudes of his peers. We therefore operate primarily between two and one-half and five years of age and strive for a small residual esotropia.

Normosensorial late-onset strabismus usually appears at approximately age three as acute or intermittent strabismus. In these cases, we prefer to wait no longer than six months. In other words, we operate relatively quickly with the objective of regaining full parallelism. It also does not seem proper to defer surgery in those children who maintain binocular vision only by use of a significant head turn or tilt, as for example in retraction syndromes or with superior oblique palsy. The same applies for intermittent exotropia worsening rapidly over short periods of time. In these cases, we operate quickly without considering the age. If the intermittency is stable, however, we wait to perform surgery until five or six years of age.

A lot has been written regarding the question of technique and gradation of surgery, such as muscle weakening or strengthening operations. One must remember that even a "weak muscle" needs only a fraction of its full strength to move the globe. What one achieves with recession/resection surgery is less a change in muscle strength than a change in the position of rest of the eyes. In a combined recession of the medial rectus and resection of the lateral rectus in the same eye, it is not the relative change in strength of these two muscles that is important, but the shift in the position of rest of the eye.

Recession, tendon lengthening, partial or total myotomy or tenotomy, myectomy, and tenectomy all are "weakening" operations. A recession is usually indicated on the recti. A similar effect can be achieved through tendon lengthening using the method of Kuhnt-Bangarter or Gonin-Hollwich.[9,68] Total myotomy or tenotomy of the rectus muscle has basically been abandoned. Partial tenotomies, specifically marginal incisions or step tenotomies (especially in reoperations), have been repopularized of late. The long-familiar adjustable suture has recently enjoyed a revival in popularity, as have traction sutures.

There is a divergence of opinion as to whether tenotomy or recession should be carried out when the oblique muscles are operated on. There are authors who always do a recession on the inferior oblique, while others do a disinsertion or myectomy near the globe. It is illuminating that a number of surgeons (Cooper, Dunlap, Dyer) have abandoned the recession and returned to tenotomy.[29,48,50] A tenotomy or tenectomy of the superior oblique tendon is recommended by Berke, or a recession (Ciancia, Haase).[14,28,58] In some cases of Brown's superior oblique syndrome, we perform a disinsertion of the muscle.

Lately, Cüppers has recommended a Faden operation (thread operation, posterior fixation suture, and retroequatorial myopexy) as a weakening procedure. Twelve to 16 mm from the original insertion, the horizontal rectus muscle is attached to the sclera by one or two sutures. In this way, a new insertion and artificial palsy are achieved which become progressively more effective on gaze to the side of the operation. This procedure is used primarily for nystagmus and for cases in which marked restriction of motility in one eye forces one to operate on the other.[38] There are clinics in which 80% of all eye muscle surgery involves a retroequatorial myopexy. Since reoperation after myopexy is difficult, it seems to me that this is a rather casual loss of later reoperation capacity. A new method for weakening a muscle has been developed by Dr. Allen Scott. He injects botulin toxin into the extraocular muscle.

"Strengthening" operations include resections, advancement, or a combination of both these procedures. Some authors will do a plication of the muscle or a "cinch" (placing of numerous sutures into the muscle to tighten them) with postoperative removal of sutures as a form of adjustment (O'Connor).[108]

With complete paresis of a muscle, for example the lateral rectus, muscle transposition of the type first popularized by Hummelsheim is recommended.[32] A portion of the superior and inferior recti is transposed to the insertion of the lateral rectus. The same can of course be done to other muscles. The Jensen procedure is similar. In this, the muscle is not severed from the globe but is split, and the lateral halves of the superior rectus and inferior rectus are connected via a suture to the appropriate halves of the lateral rectus. With total oculomotor nerve palsy, Meesmann proposed to dislocate the superior oblique out of the trochlea and transplant the muscle into the insertion of the medial rectus.[100]

Surgical technique varies among doctors, complicating discussion. The approach to the medial rectus varies among experts. The most common approach in the past was a vertical conjunctival incision halfway between the plica semilunaris and the limbus. Some authors entered Tenon's capsule at a right angle through the conjunctival incision and closed the two layers separately. Other approaches that have been recommended include incision directly at the plica (Scobee), two millimeters from the limbus (Sato), directly at the limbus (Massin), or through the fornix (Parks).[99,111125,127]

Further differences are found in the surgical technique of freeing the muscle from the muscle sheath, in severing cheek ligaments and intermuscular septa, in the site of disinsertion of the muscle, in the method of measurement, and in the placement of sutures and suture material. The differing skill levels of surgeons and the tissue characteristics of patients are additional variables.

We will now briefly discuss our current technique for the most common strabismus surgeries. We prefer a limbal incision for approach to the horizontal recti, an incision parallel to the limbus six millimeters from the vertical recti and the superior oblique, and a fornix incision for the inferior oblique. Incision at the limbus has the advantage of being relatively atraumatic. The muscle can be nicely isolated without incising Tenon's capsule. Scarring is cosmetically better than with an incision parallel but posterior to the limbus.

To recess the left medial rectus, the limbus is grasped with forceps at the conjunctiva at about 11:30 o'clock, and a radial incision of three to five millimeters is made. The conjunctiva is undermined using a spreading action of the scissors and is incised at the limbus parallel to it at 8:30 o'clock. A radial incision of three to five millimeters is made in the conjunctiva. The corners of the conjunctival flap created in this way are held with 6–0 catgut sutures placed at 10:30 and 7:30 o'clock. These serve to elevate the conjunctival flap and later to resuture it to the limbus.

The conjunctiva and Tenon's capsule are separated from the globe up to the muscle insertion via the conjunctival flap. Using blunt scissors dissection along the muscle, one separates Tenon's capsule from the sclera. A muscle hook is placed through this opening, behind the muscle, to rotate the globe. With the conjunctival flap elevated, the check ligaments, Tenon's capsule overlying the muscle, and the intermuscular membranes alongside the muscle are freed. Be careful not to injure either the muscle or the blood vessels at the muscle insertion. If the intermuscular membrane is pulled anteriorly by the first muscle hook, it should be replaced by introducing a second hook in the other direction. The first hook is then withdrawn, and the intermuscular septum is freed. The further back the muscle is freed, the more effective the recession; the less freed, the less effective the recession. Once a muscle has been adequately freed, a muscle clamp is placed two to three millimeters behind the insertion.

The muscle is severed from the sclera as flush as possible using small scissor bites. The resulting small hemorrhage points are cauterized. Three 6–0 Dexon or 6–0 vicril sutures are placed through the muscle and held with Dieffenbach clamps. The needles on these sutures are six-millimeter flat spatula needles. The muscle clamp is removed, the desired recession point is measured with calipers, and the needle is introduced into the sclera two millimeters behind the marked point. A radial scleral tunnel about two millimeters long is produced. The beginner attempts to depress the needle into the sclera. However, it is better to engage the sclera with the tip of the needle and then pull up on the needle so that it is always visible through the sclera. In this way, one is protected from perforation. After the three sutures have been placed, they are knotted three times so as not to unravel.

If an oblique (slanting) recession is desired, one should stagger the three entry points posteriorly (for example, for a recession) so that the superior entry point is three millimeters from the insertion, the middle one four millimeters, and the inferior one five millimeters away.[17,19,96]

The conjunctival flap is replaced, and the preplaced sutures are brought through the episclera and the conjunctiva at the limbus and are tied. The radial relaxing incisions are closed with interrupted sutures. The conjunctiva has to be flat at the limbus at the end of the procedure. This can be achieved by tightening the sutures.

The limbus incision for resection of the lateral rectus extends from 1:30 to about 5:30 o'clock. It is carried out as just described: The conjunctiva and Tenon's capsule are separated from the globe up to the muscle and intermuscular membrane. By spreading blunt-tipped scissors above the lateral rectus, the sclera is freed posteriorly. A muscle hook is introduced, engaging the lateral rectus. The muscle is freed of check ligaments, overlying Tenon's capsule, and intermuscular membranes. The second hook is introduced from behind and used to control freeing of the muscle. The more a muscle is freed of its connections, the less effective the resection. If one does not free the muscle from its sheath, however, the surrounding tissue is pulled

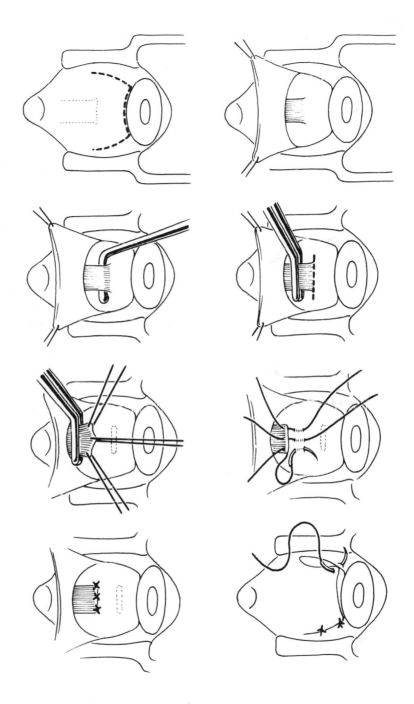

Fig. 71–Recession of a muscle (left medial rectus) with limbal incision.

forward with the resection, leading to postoperative disturbance of the anatomic relationships.

A Sattler's or Bangerter's clamp is applied to the muscle at the desired distance; for example, seven or eight millimeters from the insertion. This distance is measured with calipers without stretching the muscle. The muscle is severed between its insertion and the clamp just anterior to the original insertion. In the area where the sclera is thickest, three sutures are placed parallel to the limbus. We use 6–0 Dexon or vicril with a six-millimeter spatula needle. The scleral tunnel should be about three millimeters in length. The two needles of the double-armed central suture are passed through the middle third of the muscle one millimeter behind the muscle clamp. The two outside sutures are single armed. They are brought through the muscle, which allows the unarmed half of the suture to come around the muscle edge. The entire muscle is pulled forward with the clamp, and the knots are tied. In this way, no knots lie between muscle and sclera. The excess muscle is resected. The conjunctival flap is sutured at the limbus with catgut, silk, or adodexon sutures. With the recession, three sutures are placed vertically through the muscle tendon; with a resection, three are placed horizontally in the muscle.

For disinsertion or myectomy of the inferior oblique, the conjunctiva and Tenon's capsule are incised in the inferior temporal fornix down to the sclera. A muscle hook is placed underneath the lateral rectus, and the globe is pulled up and in. Engagement of the lateral rectus is useful for orientation. By holding up the conjunctiva-Tenon's incision, one can directly visualize the inferior oblique as a red band. A muscle hook is placed between the globe and the inferior oblique, and the tip is rotated forward to the orbital wall. The oblique is engaged by the tip of the muscle hook and is pulled up. This maneuver can also be carried out with forceps rather than a muscle hook. With direct inspection, one can assure that the muscle has not been split, leaving behind muscle fibers. The white triangle of Tenon's capsule must be visible below the inferior edge of the oblique. The hook beneath the lateral rectus is removed, and the inferior oblique is freed of attachments all the way to its insertion into the sclera. A thin curved clamp (hemostat) is applied directly at the insertion to the globe, and the muscle is severed between clamp and globe. If a clamp is not used, bleeding may result. The muscle is then freed and may be mobilized. It is replaced at its old insertion with a forceps. It is important to avoid the muscle's repositioning itself anteriorly near the insertion of the lateral or inferior rectus muscle. In this way, the muscle will readhere to the globe somewhere in its original arc of contact. If greater weakening of the inferior oblique is desired, a 0.5- to 1-centimeter excision can be done. An overeffect is not a danger. Postoperative restriction of elevation is usually due to scarring and to adhesion between the disinserted inferior oblique and the inferior rectus insertion.

Consideration should be given to the surgical findings. The position of the eye under anesthesia pre- and postoperatively should be noted, especially when the two globes do not have the same position. This is dependent in part on the depth of anesthesia. The appearance of straight eyes should not fool one into doing too little. Passive movement of the globes, the so-called "forced duction test," is important. This must be done prior to surgical intervention and should be repeated after severing the muscle. One should look for anatomic anomalies, for example, broad insertions or increased rigidity of a muscle. Intraoperative problems such as heavy bleeding should be noted.

There is a question about the amount of required surgery, beginning with the degree of deviation. All possible combinations exist between those surgeons who do not measure the angle at all and those who are most exact in angle measurements and millimeters operated.

It would seem reasonable for comparative purposes to measure the angle of deviation as exactly as possible. One must indicate the method used, however (corneal reflex, synoptophore, alternating prism cover test, or simultaneous prism cover test).

Furthermore, it must be remembered that the angle is not stable but is variable. This is true in the immediate preoperative period, with variations according to the time of day, fatigue, and general health of the patient. It is also true over long periods of time, for esotropia tends to decrease and exotropia tends to increase.

Before one discusses the exact millimeter dosages, one should consider that the average globe radius is about 75 mm. Five degrees of rotation are equivalent to one millimeter. One has to move a muscle pair by one millimeter — for example, the medial rectus recession of one millimeter and advancement of the lateral rectus one millimeter — to shift the globe's position of rest by five degrees of divergence. This is if the muscle is the sole mechanical determinant of the position of rest, without considering the effects of Tenon's capsule, the check ligaments, and blood supplies to the globe.

Various formulas exist for the exact ratios employed in eye muscle surgery, the best known of which is that of Alvaro: three degrees of esotropia are corrected by each millimeter of recession.[4] This should result in a correction of 12 degrees with four millimeters of recession. Resection of the lateral rectus gives 1.5 degrees of effect per millimeter. Resection of seven millimeters would give a correction of 10.5 degrees. Combining recession and resection increases the effect by 20%. Recession of the medial rectus of four millimeters combined with resection of the lateral rectus of seven millimeters would give an overall correction of 27 degrees.

Other authors start with the total amount of muscle upon which one has operated. The amount of recession resection is added and then multiplied by an experience factor that usually varies between one and two degrees per millimeter. A recession of four millimeters combined with a resection of seven millimeters equals an overall surgical total of 11 mm. If the experience value is 1.5 degrees per millimeter, the expected correction is 16.5 degrees. If the experience factor is two degrees per millimeter, a correction of 22 degrees is obtained.

The following formula, combining the experience of a number of ophthalmology departments, was presented at the International Congress of Ophthalmology in Munich:

$$\text{Correction} = 2 \text{ times resection} + 5 \text{ times}$$
$$\text{recession} - 12[115]$$

One other eye clinic had the following formula:

$$\text{Correction} = 2 \text{ times resection} + 5 \text{ times}$$
$$\text{recession} - 22$$

According to these formulas, a recession of four millimeters and a resection of seven millimeters would achieve 22 degrees of correction in the first case, but only 12 degrees in the second.

According to Cüppers, the relationship between recession and resection should be 1:2 for esotropia and exotropia. With angles of more than 20 degrees, the relationship should increase to 1:2.5. The angle of correction is calculated according to the diameter of the globe. With an average diameter of 24 mm, it is four degrees 42 minutes per millimeter; with a globe diameter of 21.3 mm, it is 5 degrees 23 minutes per millimeter; and with a diameter of 18 mm, it is 6 degrees 22 minutes per millimeter.

A recession of three millimeters combined with a resection of six millimeters with a globe diameter of 21.3 mm would give a correction of 16 degrees.[37] Many surgeons have a standard procedure that they vary according to their own experience to the size of the angle of deviation. We ourselves begin with the most common angle of 15 degrees and perform either a recession of four millimeters combined with a resection of six to seven millimeters or a recession of both medial rectus muscles by four to four and one-half millimeters. With smaller angles, we use slightly less surgery; with greater angles, more surgery. Should only one eye be operated upon (recession resection), or should surgery be symmetrically divided between both eyes (bimedial recession)? Should correction be obtained in one sitting or in stages? All viewpoints have their defenders. The divergence of opinion is so extreme that some surgeons will operate upon only one muscle per surgery, while others may operate upon as many as four horizontal and two oblique muscles or two recti and four oblique muscles at the same time.

Every honest surgeon will admit that his results vary. The variation is sometimes surprisingly great, for which no explanation can be found despite standardization of one's surgical technique and careful evaluation of each case. The variation and results may be greater the more examiners and the more surgeons involved. One cause of such clutter is intrinsic to each gradation formula: The closer one comes to one's goal, the greater the danger that one achieves overcorrection. If one wants to be most correct for any individual case, the solution is not heterogeneous statistics but the careful differentiation of each case.

It is therefore not possible to set up simple inviolable rules. Certain guidelines are possible, however. Surgery should not be too extreme, and only in rare cases for purely cosmetic reasons should one accept postoperative restriction of motility. This means that one cannot recess or resect excessively if a functional goal is in mind. On the average, recession of the medial rectus should not be more than five millimeters; a resection of the lateral rectus, not more than eight to ten millimeters. Greater surgery is allowable depending upon the size of the globe and the distance that the muscle insertion is from the limbus. The degrees of surgery are especially important with combined operations. Surgery on only one horizontal muscle is usually futile even with heterophorias.[52] Roughly every fourth operation has an unexpected result.[137] Exotropia requires more extensive surgery than esotropia of the same degree. Vertical surgery on the vertical elevators and depressors must be graded carefully. In vertical surgery, an isolated recession or resection has a significantly greater effect than with the horizontal recti. In contrast, tenotomy of the superior oblique or myectomy of the inferior oblique can be carried out without danger of a significant loss of these muscle functions. Each case must be differentiated as much as possible. Only very similar cases may be combined for comparison. Differentiation into "A" and "V" patterns, the congenital squint syndrome, normosensorial late-onset strabismus, strabismus sursoadductorius, and dissociated vertical deviation is important. For example, with a congenital "V" pattern strabismus of 15 to 20 degrees, we proceed differently (vertical offset inferiorly and recession of both medial recti, and possible myectomy of both inferior obliques) than with normal sensorial late-onset strabismus of the same degree (unilateral recession resection).

Since a degree of uncertainty is present with strabismus surgery, it is best to warn parents and patients about the possibility of the need for more than one surgical procedure. On one hand, there is the risk of regression to the old angle of deviation with insufficient surgery, especially with deep-rooted anomalous retinal correspondence. To avoid this, we use graded occlusion during the postoperative period. On the other hand, the cosmetically undesirable secondary exotropia, possibly with parodoxic diplopia, can develop with excessive surgery, amblyopia of one eye, and muscular insufficiency. For those puzzling cases that despite careful preoperative measurements evolve into postoperative exotropia, one has to remember that there are cases of esotropia that spontaneously convert to consecutive exotropia over time. Unfortunately, we have insufficient criteria currently to be able to avoid this problem.

With exotropia, it is also to be expected that over time the motor position of rest will become more divergent. One may therefore have to reoperate at a later point in time.

Paraphrasing Hippocrates, who said "the art is difficult, the right moment hard to grasp, and life is long," we can say that the surgical indication and gradation are difficult, the surgical technique is easy, and the life expectancy of our small strabismus patients is long.

THERAPY FOR DISORDERS OF BINOCULAR VISION

It is useful to differentiate between those cases in which one is able to achieve normal binocular vision and those in which this is not possible.

Normal binocular vision that is "restitutio ad integrum"—truly normal binocular vision or a true cure — is achieved only in those patients who had developed true binocular vision by the second or third year of life, prior to the relatively late onset of their strabismus. In this group are included normosensorial late-onset strabismus, fully accommodative strabismus, and intermittent exotropia.

Normosensorial late-onset strabismus was discussed previously. For example, a three-year-old without previous history of eye problems suddenly develops strabismus. The deviation is intermittent at first and then constant. Sometimes the child admits to diplopia or closes the deviating eye. The angle will increase rapidly over a short period of time. Presumably, there was preexisting esophoria, which is now decompensated. Significant hyperopia is not present, or its correction does not help.

These cases should be operated on as quickly as possible, at least within six months after onset of the strabismus. If one waits longer, suppression develops, which may hinder fusion later on. Occasionally, prisms need to be prescribed as well. We use alternate occlusion postoperatively to avoid relapse of the strabismus. Occlusion is interrupted twice a day, morning and afternoon, for one half-hour to encourage binocular vision and parallelism.

Fully accommodative strabismus with straight eyes for distance and glasses for near gaze requires no other treatment than the wearing of glasses. This should be instituted immediately after onset of the esotropia. Intermittent exotropia also belongs in this group. Basic exodeviation at a distance of more than eight to ten degrees is an indication for surgery. Surgery should not be unduly delayed, because suppression of the foveal region of the deviated eye can occur. This may later be detrimental to the achievement of straight eyes, as in the sense of horror fusionis. We operate as soon as the child threatens to become manifest for both distance and near gaze.

The same is true for "A" and "V" patterns or paralysis, where binocular vision is maintained through head position in a certain direction.

A partial normalization in cases of accommodative esotropia with convergence excess is possible by changing the accommodation/convergence ratio. In certain cases, parallelism for distance and near gaze can be achieved using bifocals.

TREATMENT WITH ANOMALOUS RETINAL CORRESPONDENCE

Treatment of anomalous retinal correspondence requires considerable therapy, with many visits for orthoptics. Using the Synoptophore, central retinal areas are stimulated to return to normal retinal correspondence. Peripheral areas, however, are not affected. After long training on the synoptophore, normal binocular vision is sometimes achieved by the patient.

Vision in free space differs considerably from vision at the synoptophore. If after completion of orthoptic treatment, a manifest deviation that is not correctable with prisms is still present in free space viewing, one can be certain that normal binocular vision is not present. Either there is normal retinal correspondence that can only be elicited on the synoptophore, or strong suppression or anomalous retinal correspondence, or both, is still present. A simple treatment of and prophylaxis against anomalous retinal correspondence is total alternating occlusion over a period of years.

If one checks the results of treatment of anomalous retinal correspondence with simple tests such as the cover test and Bagolini lenses, one rarely finds a truly complete fuser. This statement applies to all known treatments. Treatment methods are based on the concept that anomalous retinal correspondence is a sensory adaptation to the strabismus, and that this sensory abnormality can be returned to normal. With microstrabismus, however, we have seen that a predilection for anomalous retinal correspondence is probably inherited. This justifies modification of our previous thinking. We have reported on our experience of treating anomalous retinal correspondence with penalization. It has turned out that our expectations for this method of therapy were too optimistic, however, and that normalization of anomalous retinal correspondence with penalization is not to be achieved.

Lately, surgical and prismatic overcorrection into resultant exotropia has been recommended for treatment of anomalous retinal correspondence. We are highly skeptical of this. Every ophthalmologist is familiar with cases of surgically produced consecutive exotropia without normalization of the anomalous retinal correspondence. We think it is more practical in cases of anomalous retinal correspondence to seek microesotropia. This leads, in our opinion, to functional binocularity. It is admittedly not ideal but protects one from secondary exotropia.

Many authors are of the opinion that anomalous retinal correspondence can be eliminated by means of exercises. Here too we are reticent. Binocular vision with anomalous retinal correspondence usually develops spontaneously. Energetic therapy may cause damage. This is because antisuppression measures may lead to asthenopic symptoms and complaints of diplopia.[33]

This naturally raises the question of what is left of orthoptic treatment if one abandons efforts at reeducating abnormal retinal correspondence. We emphasize here that our viewpoint is that of the practicing ophthalmologist. Orthoptic clinics in eye departments concerned with education and research may be a different situation. Here too, however, emphasis has shifted from therapy to diagnosis.

The orthoptist has a number of important functions in the ophthalmic practice which make this a most worthwhile and interesting profession. Children today are brought to the ophthalmologist much earlier. Preschool vision checks, orthoptic examinations, treatment and supervision of patching, and communication about the condition with the parents can be done by the orthoptist, and this relieves the ophthalmologist of a great deal of work. After surgery, exercises are often necessary.

Traffic accidents, which are accompanied by increased orbital trauma and disturbances of fusion with cerebral contusions, bring new problems to the ophthalmologist. In this instance, the orthoptist can be useful. If in addition the orthoptist performs visual field examinations, participates in the recording of clinical history, and occasionally assists with strabismus surgery, he truly has a satisfying career. Too much treatment with instruments or unrealistic expectations for therapy serve neither the orthoptist, the patient, nor the ophthalmologist.

Generally, it must be said that the theoretical basis for binocular vision still has large gaps. Until these are filled, therapy is not on firm grounds. It is therefore not surprising that for many therapeutic questions there is no "unite de doctrine."

The goal and intensity of therapy differ from ophthalmologist to ophthalmologist. New recommendations constantly arise, with increasingly greater promise for success. After years, however, they are replaced by other methods.

A "look backward" justifies a certain skepticism. One hundred and fifty years ago, the first wave of surgical enthusiasm predicted the ability to eliminate strabismus and amblyopia with surgery. Overcorrection, possibly with paralysis of the medial rectus, is now again recommended for normalization of anomalous retinal correspondence.[40] One should remember that after medial rectus tenotomy, there have always developed undesired secondary exotropias that did not heal.

The prismatic treatment method of Sattler has also been revived, with cure rates as high as 95%, independent of the type of strabismus.[13,117] Sattler himself approached his therapy method primarily from the concept of normal sensorial late-onset strabismus.[126] Other authors cite very high success ratios with esotropia simply through the constant full correction of hyperopia.[121] Instrument exercises with various modifications for treatment of anomalous retinal correspondence have achieved differing reputations over time. A skeptical attitude is certainly in order whenever an alleged treatment method is recommended that does not differentiate the special types of strabismus treated. One should also not be too impressed by preliminary reports of favorable therapy and unrealistically high success rates. One should wait and allow these to be based upon solid statistics. It is interesting to learn the latest methods. It is more important, however, to know which methods have already been abandoned. It is most useful to know which methods are still valid, having proven themselves over time.

It is to be hoped that new knowledge will bring new therapeutic successes. Here, too, each physician will benefit by reviewing his own cases to obtain his own verdict. Therapy must be selective, and the effort must be worthwhile. The doctor, the parents, and the small patients should be spared going in false directions.

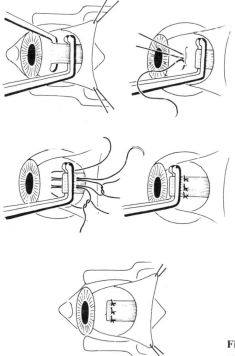

Fig. 72–Resection of a muscle (left lateral rectus) with limbal incision.

References

1. Abraham, S.V., The use of miotics in the treatment of convergent strabismus. Am. J. Ophth. *32*, 233–240 (1949).
2. Abraham, S.V., Bilateral ametropic amblyopia. J. Pediat. Ophth. *1*, 57–61 (1964).
3. Adelstein, F. und Cüppers, C., Zum Problem der echten und der scheinbaren Abducenslähmung (Das sogenannte "Blokkierungssyndrom"). Klin. Mbl. Augenhk. *46. Beiheft*, 271–278 (1966).
4. Alvaro, M.E., Simultaneous Surgical Correction of Vertical and Horizontal Deviation. Ophthalmologica *120*, 191–197 (1950).
5. Anderson, J.R., Causes and treatment of congenital eccentric nystagmus. Br. J. Ophth. *37*, 267 (1953).
6. Andrée, G., Zur Entwicklung der foveolaren Fixation, 66. Ber. dtsch. Ophthalm. Ges. 271–273 (1964).
7. Bagolini, B., Tecnica per l'esame della visione binoculare senza introduzione di elementi dissocianti "Test del vetro striato." Boll. Ocul. *37*, 195–209 (1958).
8. Bagshaw, J., The "Heavy Eye" Phenomenon. Brit. orthopt. J. *23*, 75–78 (1966).
9. Bamert, W., Erfahrung mit der Sehnenverlängerung nach Kuhnt-Bangerter. Ophthalmologica *131*, 257–261 (1956).
10. Bangerter, A., Die Okklusion in der Pleoptik und Orthoptik. Klin. Mbl. Augenhk. *136*, 305–331 (1960).
11. Bangerter, A., Amblyopiebehandlung. Karger, Basel (1955).
12. Baumann, H.E., Die Anwendung des Polatests in der Praxis. Ophthalmologica *158*, 612–621 (1969).
13. Bérard, P.V., Les prismes en thérapeutique ophthalmologique. Bull. Soc. Ophthal. France *4* (1965).
14. Berke, R.N., Surgical treatment of hypertropia. Strabismus Symposium. New Orleans, 190–230, C.V. Mosby, St. Louis (1962).
15. Bielschowsky, A., Das Einwärtsschielen der Myopen. 43. Ber. Dtsch. Ophthalm. Ges., 245–248 (1922).
16. Bielschowsky, A., Die einseitigen und gegensinnigen (dissoziierten Vertikalbewegungen der Augen. Graefes-Arch. Ophth. *124*, 493–512 (1930).
17. Bietti, G.B., Su un accorgimento tecnico (recessione e reinserzione obliqua a ventaglio dei muscoli retti orizzontali) per la correzione di atteggiamenti a V o A di grado modesti negli strabismi concomitanti. Boll. Ocul. *49*, 581–588 (1970).
18. Binder, H.F. *et al.*, The red filter treatment of excentric fixation. Amer. J. Orthopt. *13*, 64 (1963).
19. Boyd, T.A.S., Leitch, G.T., and Budd, G.E., A new treatment for A and V patterns in strabismus by slanting muscle insertions. A preliminary report. Can. J. Ophth. *6*, 170 (1971).
20. Brown, H.W., The superior obl. tendon sheath syndrom. Strabismus Ophthalmic Symposium I. ed Allen, J.H.–C.V. Mosby Company, St. Louis (1950).
21. Brown, E.V.L., Net average yearly changes in refraction of atropinized eyes from birth to beyond middle life. Arch. Ophth. *19*, 719 (1938).
22. De Buffon, G.L.L., Sur la cause du strabisme ou des yeux louches. Memoires de l'académie royale des sciences, 321–345 (1748).
23. Burian, H.M., Use of bifocal spectacles in the treatment of accommodative esotropia. Brit. orth. J. *13*, 3–6 (1956).
24. Burian, H.M., Exodeviations: their classification, diagnosis, and treatment. Am. J. Ophth. *62*, 1161 (1966).
25. Burian, H. und Miller, J.E., Comitant convergent strabismus with acute onset. Am. J. Ophth. *45*, 55–64 (1958).
26. Ciancia, A.O., Sensorial Relationship in A and V syndromes. Transact. Ophth. Soc. Unit. Kingdom. *82*, 243–251 (1962).

27. Ciancia, A.O., Management of esodeviations under the age of two. Int. Ophthalm. Clinics, Strabismus, 503–518 (1966).

28. Ciancia, A.O. y Diaz, J.P., Retroceso del oblicuo superior Primeros resultados. Arch. Oftal. B. Ares XLV, *45*, 193–200 (1970).

29. Cooper, E.L. and Sandall, G.S., Recession versus free myotomie at the insertion of the inferior oblique muscle. J. pediatric. ophthalmol. *6*, 6–10 (1969).

30. Costenbader, F.D., Early surgery of strabismus. Arch. Ophth. Chicago *71*, 761 (1964).

31. Costenbader, F.D., Symposium: The "A" and "V" Patterns in Strabismus. Transactions Am. of Ophthalmol. and Otolaryn. *68*, 3 (1964).

32. Crone, R.A., Alternating Hyperphoria. Brit. J. Ophthalm. *38*, 591 (1954).

33. Crone, R.A. und van den Bosch, I.G., The sweet and bitter fruits of orthoptic exercise. Perspectives in Ophthalmology II. Excerpta Medica Monograph, 171–178 (1970).

34. Cüppers, C., Moderne Schielbehandlung. Klin. Mbl. Augenhk. *129*, 579–604 (1956).

35. Cüppers, C., Grenzen und Möglichkeiten der pleoptischen Therapie. Klin. Mbl. Augenhk. *38*, 33 (1961).

36. Cüppers, C., Some reflections on the possibility of influencing the pathological fixation act. Ann. roy. Coll. Surg. Engl. *38*, 308–325 (1966).

37. Cüppers, C., Korrektur der Horizontalabweichung. BVA Arbeitskreis Schielbehandlung, Wiesbaden 1972, *5*, 11–19 (1973).

38. Cüppers, C., The so-called "Fadenoperation." Second ISA congress Marseille 1974, Kimpton (im Druck).

39. Cüppers, C. and Mühlendyck, H., Die Entwicklung der Amblyopietherapie unter dem Gesichtspunkt der Gießener Klinik. Second ISA congress Marseille 1974, Kimpton (im Druck).

40. De Decker, W., Holzki, U. and Laube, U., Behandlung der anomalen Korrespondenz durch artifizielle Sekundärdivergenz. Ophthalmologica *157*, 142–153 (1969).

41. Deller, M. und Brack, B., Le traitement chirurgical de choix des ésotropies obliques en V. Ophthalmologica *161*, 340–345 (1970).

42. Deller, M. und Brack, B., Nouveau procédé de traitement de l'amblyopie strabique à fixation excentrique. Ophthalmologica *160*, 152 (1970).

43. Dieffenbach, J.F., Über das Schielen und die Heilung desselben durch die Operation. Berlin (1842).

44. Doden, W. und Bunge, H., Fusionsstörungen nach Schädelhirntraumen. Klin. Mbl. Augenhk. *146*, 846–853 (1965).

45. Donders, F.C., Die Anomalien der Refraktion und der Akkommodation des Auges. Wien (1866).

46. Duane, A., A new classification of the motor anomalies of the eye. New York, J.H. Vaio and Co. (1897).

47. Duane, A., Congenital deficiency of abduction, associated with impairment of abduction, retraction movements, contractions of the palpebral fissure and oblique movements of the eye. Arch. Ophth. *34*, 133–159 (1905).

48. Dunlap, E.A., Inferior oblique weakening. Annals Ophthal. *4*, 905 (1972).

49. Dunlap, E.A., Vertical displacement of horizontal recti. Symposium on Strabismus, New Orleans, 307–330, C.V. Mosby, St. Louis (1971).

50. Dyer, J.A., Tenotomy of the inferior oblique muscle at its scleral insertion. Arch. Ophthalmol. *68*, 176 (1962).

51. Esslen, E. und Papst, W., Die Bedeutung der Elektromyographie für die Analyse von Motilitätsstörungen der Augen. Karger, Basel (1961).

52. Foster, J., Pemberton, E.C. and Freedman, C., Graded squint operation. Trans. Opht. Soc. Unit. Kingdom *62*, 320 at 329 (1942).

53. Franceschetti, A. und Bischler, V., Strabisme concomitant aigu chez l'adulte. Confinia neurologica (1947–1948).

54. Gobin, M., Anteroposition of the inferior Oblique Muscle in V-Esotropia. Ophthalmologica *148*, 325–341 (1964).

55. Goldmann, H., Gedanken eines Nicht-Strabologen zur Pathophysiologie des optischen Raumsinnes. Docum. Ophthal. *23*, 101–107 (1967).

56. Goldschmidt, M., Beitrag zur Anatomie des Musculus rectus externus und des Musculus rectus internus bei Hund und Mensch. Ophthalmologica *157*, 381–390 (1969).

57. Haase, H.J., Binoculare Korrektion. Zeitschr. Optometrie (1959).

58. Haase, W., Zur operativen Behandlung horizontaler Inkomitanz im Rahmen des frühkindlichen Strabismus (A-Syndrom). Klin. Mbl. Augenhk. *160*, 648–662 (1972).

59. Hamburger, F.A., Horror Fusionis. 54. Beiheft der Klin. Mbl. Augenhk. (1970).

60. Harms, H., Ort und Wesen der Bildhemmung bei Schielenden. Graefes Arch. Ophth. *138*, 149–209 (1937).

61. Helveston, E.M. und von Noorden, G.K., Microtropia. Arch. Ophthal. *78*, 272–281 (1967).

62. Hess, W.R., Eine neue Untersuchungsmethode bei Doppelbildern. Arch. Augenhk. 62, 233–238 (1960).

63. Hirschberg, J., Beiträge zur Lehre vom Schielen und von der Schieloperation. Zbl. prakt. Augenhk. *10*, 5–9 (1886).

64. Hoeve, J. van der, Amblyopia and squint, escape squint. Docum. ophthal. *392*, 7–8 (1954).

65. Hofmann, F.B. und Bielschowsky, A., Die Verwertung der Kopfneigung zur Diagnostik von Augenmuskellähmungen aus der Heber- und Senkergruppe. Graefes Arch. Ophth. *51*, 174 bis 185 (1900).

66. Holland, G., Häufigkeit und Vorkommen der anomalen Netzhautkorrespondenz. Graefes Arch. Ophth. *166*, 556–582 (1964).

67. Holland, G., Die anomale Korrespondenz als erworbene bzw. angeborene, zum Teil familiär auftretende Anomalie. 65. Ber. Dtsch. Ophthal. Ges., 471–474 (1963).

68. Hollwich, F., Die Sehnenverlängerung nach Gonin. Ophthalmologica *142*, 412 (1961).

68a. Hotchkiss, M.G., Miller, N.R. Clark, A.W. et al, Bilateral Duane's retraction syndrome. Arch. Ophthalmol. *98*, 870–874 (1980).

69. Hubel, D.H. und Wiesel, T.N., Binocular interaction in striate cortex of kittens reared with artificial squint. J. Neurophys. *28*, 1060 (1965).

70. Huber, A., Die Miotica in der Behandlung des Strabismus concomitans. Ophthalmologica *127*, 362–367 (1954).

71. Hugonnier, R. und Magnard, P., Les déséquilibres oculomoteurs observés en cas de myopie forte. Ann. Oculist. (Paris) *202*, 713–724 (1969).

72. Hummelsheim, E., Über Sehnentransplantation am Auge. Ber. Dtsch. Ophthal. Ges. *34*, 248–252 (1907).

73. Jampolsky, A., The prism test for strabismus screening. J. pediat. Ophthalm. *1*, 30–34 (1964).

74. Jampolsky, A., Flom, M. und Thorson, J.C., Membrane fresnel prisms — A new therapeutic device. Second ISA congress. Acapulco (1970).

75. Jampolsky, A., The A and V syndromes. Symposium. New Orleans, 157–177, C.V. Mosby, St. Louis (1962).

76. Kestenbaum, A., Nouvelle opération du nystagmus. Bull. Soc. Ophthal. Fr. *6*, 599 (1953).

77. Kettesy, A., Bifokalbrille gegen konvergentes Begleitschielen. Klin. Mbl. Augenhk. *141*, 209–217 (1962).

78. Knapp, Ph., The surgical treatment of double elevator paralysis. Trans. Amer. Ophth. Soc. *67*, 304–323 (1969).

79. Knapp, Ph., Vertically incomitant horizontal strabismus the so-called A and V syndrome. Trans. Am. Ophth. Soc. *57*, 666 (1959).

80. Krewson, W., Secondary functions of the inferior oblique muscle. Arch. Ophth. Chicago *44*, 158–160 (1950).

81. Lancaster, W.B., Terminology in ocular motility and allied subjects. Am. J. Ophth. *26*, 122–132 (1943).

82. Lang, J., Zur praktischen Bedeutung der anomalen Netzhautkorrespondenz. Ophthalmologica *133*, 215–217 (1957).

83. Lang, J., Über die Amblyopie ohne Schielen und bei unauffälligem Schielwinkel. Ophthalmologica *141*, 429–434 (1961).

84. Lang, J., Fixationsflucht, Photophobie und Strabismus, in Disorders of Ocular Motility, Symposion DOG 1977 Freiburg G. Kommerell, Bergmann München, 1978, 307–310.

85. Lang, J., Evaluation in Small Angle Strabismus or Microtropia. Strabism. Symp. Gießen (1966). Karger, Basel, 219–222 (1968).

86. Lang, J., Die Bedeutung des primären Mikrostrabismus für die Entstehung des Schielens. Klin. Mbl. Augenhk. *151*, 352 bis 361 (1967).

87. Squint dating from birth or with early onset. Transactions First International Congress of Orthoptists, 231–237, 1968, Kimpton, London.

87a. Lang, J. A New Hypothesis on Latent Nystagmus and on the Congenital Squint Syndrome. Docum. Opthal. Proc. Series, Vol. 32 ed by A.Th.M. van Balen & W.A. Houtman 1982, Dr. W. Junk Publishers, The Hague.

88. Lang, J., Welche Schielfälle können geheilt werden? Ophthalmologica *156*, 190–196 (1968).

89. Lang, J., Microtropia. Arch. Ophth., Chicago *81*, 758–762 (1969).

90. Lang, J., Einfache Differentialdiagnostik und gezielte Behandlung des Strabismus convergens. Klin. Mbl. Augenhk. *155*, 457–475 (1969).

91. Lang, J., Speiser, P., Witmer, R. und Jost, P., Geheilte Schielamblyopie: Normales Binokularsehen oder Alternieren? Ophthalmologica *154*, 76–80 (1967).

92. Lang, J. und Würth, A., Photographic representation of anomalous correspondence. Ophthal. Res. *1*, 88–93 (1970).

93. Lang, J. Zur Anwendung der Ausschleichokklusion. Klin. Mbl. Augenhk. *160*, 688–693 (1972).

94. Lang, J. Mikrostrabismus, 2. erweiterte Auflage, 64. Beiheft, Bücherei des Augenarztes, Enke Stuttgart, 1982.

95. Lang, J., Der Treffversuch zur Prüfung des stereoskopischen Sehens. Klin. Mbl. Augenhk. *165*, 895–897 (1974).

96. Lavat, J. et Bons, G., Reculs obliques dans la chirurgie des syndromes A. et V. Bull. Soc. Ophth. *3*, 317–320 (1972).

97. Locket, N.A., The dual nature of human extra-ocular muscle. Brit. J. Orthopt. *25*, 2–11 (1968).

98. Lyle, T.K. und Bridgeman, G.J.O., Worth and Chavasse's Squint. Ninth Edition. Bailliere, Tindall & Cox, London (1959).

99. Massin, M. und Hudelo, J., L'incision de la conjonctive au limbe dans les operations pour strabisme et pour décollement de rétine. Ann. ocul. Paris, 995–1003 (1962).

100. Meesmann, A., Über die Trochlearisüberpflanzung bei totaler angeborener Okulomotoriusparalyse. Klin. Mbl. Augenhk. *135*, 247–252 (1959).

101. Mein, J., Clinical features of the retraction syndrome. Transactions of the First international Congress of Orthopists, 165–177, Kimpton, London (1968).

102. Miller, J.E., Vertical recti transplantation in the A and V syndromes. Arch. Ophth. *64*, 175 (1960).

103. Minkowsky, M., Über frühzeitige Bewegungen, Reflexe und Reaktionen des menschlichen Foetus und ihre Beziehungen zum foetalen Nerven- und Muskelsystem. Schweiz. med. Wschr. *Bd. 3*, 721–724 (1922).

104. Moore, S., The action of diisoprophylfluorphosphate in the management of esotropia. The First international Congress of Orthopists. Kimpton, London, 358–360 (1967).

105. Paliaga, G.P., A. Ghisolfi, G. Giunta et A. Decarli: Rotations oculaires et reflets cornéens. Ophthalmologica 181:231–236 (1980).

106. Müller, P., Über das Sehen der Amblyopen. Ophthalmologica *121*, 143–149 (1951).

107. von Noorden, G.K. und Maumenee, A.E., Clinical observations on stimulus-deprivation amblyopia (Amblyopia ex anopsia). Amer. J. Ophthal. *65*, 220–224 (1968).

108. O'Connor, R., The Cinch Operation. Brit. J. Ophth. *39*, 495–502 (1955).
109. Ogle, K.N., Fixation disparity and fusional processes in binocular single vision. Am. J. Ophth. *36*, 1063–1087 (1949).
110. Panum, P.L., Physiologische Untersuchungen über das Sehen mit zwei Augen. Kiel, Schwersche Buchhandlung (1858).
111. Parks, M., Fornix incision for horizontal rectus muscle surgery. Am. J. Ophth. *65*, (1968).
112. Parks, M. und Eustis, A.T., Monofixational phoria. Am. orth. J. *11*, 38–45 (1961).
113. Parks, M.M., The monofixational syndrome. Trans. Am. Ophth. Soc. *67*, 609 (1969).
114. Pfandl, E., Ein neuer Weg zur Verhinderung der Ausbildung einer ANK beim Strab. conc. Acta XVIII, Concil. Ophth. Belgia *1*, 202 (1958).
115. Pietruschka, G., Kombinierte Myektomie und Rücklagerung bei Strabismus convergens. 20. Concilium Ophth. Germania, Acta 621–626 (1966).
116. Pigassou, R. und Garipuy, J., Traitement de la fixation excentrique par le port d'un prisme et l'occlusion. Bull. Soc. Franc. Ophthal. *79*, 367 (1966).
117. Pigassou, R. und Garipuy, J., Traitement du strabisme dans l'espace libre. Arch. opht., Paris *26*, 445–458 (1966).
118. Plenck, J.J., Doctrina de morbis oculorum, Vienna (1777).
119. Pouliquen, P., Zum Problem der Penalisation. Klin. Mbl. Augenhk. *161*, 130 (1972).
120. Quéré, M.A., Die Methoden der Penalisation in der Behandlung des Strabismus convergens. Klin. Mbl. Augenhk. *161*, 140 (1972).
121. Réthy, St. und Gal, S., Ergebnisse der konservativen Schielbehandlung durch Überkorrektur der manifesten Hypermetropie. Klin. Mbl. Augenhk. *150*, 170–180 (1967).
122. Richter, S., Untersuchung über die Heredität des Strabismus concomitans. VEB Georg Thieme *35*, (1967) (Monographie).
123. Roper-Hall, M.J. and Roper-Hall, G., The superior oblique click syndrom. Orthoptics, Sec. int. Orth. Congress, 360–366 (1971).
124. Rubin, W., Reverse Prism and calibrated occlusion. Am. J. ophth. *59*, 271 (1965).
125. Sato, O., Measuring for recession operations from the limbal conjunctiva. Strabismus 69. Trans. Consilium Europaeum, London 1969, Henry Kimpton.
126. Sattler, C.H., Über die Behandlung des Schielens und über die Bedeutung der Prismenbrillen für die Wiederherstellung des beidäugigen Sehaktes. Klin. Mbl. Augenhk. *105*, 182–190 (1940).
127. Scobee, R.G., The oculorotory muscles. The C.V. Mosby Company, St. Louis (1952).
128. Sevrin, G. und De Corte, H., Surgery for eccentric fixation displacement. Strabismus Symp. Gießen (1966). Karger, Basel/New York, 89–97 (1968).
129. Slapater, F.J., Age norms of refraction and vision. Arch. Ophth. *43*, 466–481 (1950).
130. Steidele, M., Die Grundschulung bei Amblyopie in der Pleoptik- und Orthoptikschule St. Gallen. Zehnder, St. Gallen (1962).
131. Stilling, J., Untersuchungen über die Entstehung der Kurzsichtigkeit (1887).
132. Swan, K.C., The blind spot mechanism in Strabismus. Strabismus ophthalmic Symp. II, 201–211. C.V. Mosby Comp. ed Allen, J.H., St. Louis (1958).
133. Türk, Bemerkungen zu einem Fall von Retraktionsbewegungen des Auges. Zbl. Augenhk. *23*, 14–18 (1899).
134. Urist, M.J., Horizontal squint with secondary vertical deviations. Arch. Ophth. *46*, 245 (1951).
135. Urrets-Zavalia, A., Paralisis bilateral congenital del musculo oblicuo inferior. Arch. oftal., Buenos Aires *23*, 182 (1948).
136. Wilczek, M., Neue Methode zur Untersuchung der anomalen Netzhautkorrespondenz. Klin. Mbl. Augenhk. *145*, 882–887 (1964).
137. Ward, B.A., The functional results in cases of convergent squint. Am. J. Ophth. *58*, 258–261 (1964).
138. Ward, B.A., The heavy eye phenomenon. Trans. ophthal. Soc. Unit. Kingdom *87*, 717–726 (1967).

139. Willi, H., Das Phänomen der untergehenden Sonne beim Neugeborenen. Ann. paediat. (Basel), _174_, 87 (1950), _178_, 312 (1952).

140. Worth, Claud: Squint, its causes, pathology and treatment. John Bale. London 1903, p. 29.

Suggested Reading

Arruga, A., Diagnostico y Tratamiento del Estrabismo. C. Bermeyo, Madrid (1958).

Aust, W., Pleoptik und Orthoptik. S Karger, Basel (1966).

Bielschowsky, A., Lectures on Motor Anomalies. Dartmouth Publications, Hanover, New Hampshire (1956).

Bredemeyer, H.G. und Bullock, K., Orthoptics. The C.V. Mosby Company, St. Louis (1968).

Burian, H.M. and von Noorden, G.K., Binocular Vision and Ocular Motility. The C.V. Mosby Company, St. Louis (1974).

Cashell, G.T. und Durran, I.M., Handbook of Orthoptic Principles. E. & S. Livingstone, London (1967).

Castanera, A., Nistagmus Ocular. Editorial Paz Montalvo, Madrid (1963).

Ciancia, A.O., Las secuelas sensoriales del Estrabismo. Macchi, Buenos Aires (1960).

Crone, R.A., Diplopia. Excerpta Medica, Amsterdam (1973).

Duke-Elder, St., System of Ophthalmology, Vol. VI, Ocular Motility and Strabismus. Henry Kimpton, London (1973).

Fink, W.H., Surgery of the Vertical Muscles of the Eye. Charles C. Thomas, Springfield (1962).

Folk, E.R., Treatment of Strabismus. Charles C. Thomas, Springfield (1965).

Hamburger, F.A., Stellungsanomalien. In: Der Augenarzt. Bd. III, Thieme, Leipzig (1960).

Hugonnier, R. und S., Strabismes. Masson et Cie., Paris (1965).

Keiner, G.B.J., New Viewpoints on the Origin of Squint. Martinus Nijhoff, The Hague (1951).

Krüger, K.E., Physiologische und methodische Grundlagen der Pleoptik und Orthoptik. VEB Georg Thieme, Leipzig (1967).

Lyle, T.K. und Bridgeman, G.J.O., Worth and Chavasse's Squint. Ninth Edition. Bailliere, Tindall & Cox, London (1959).

Lyle, T.K. und Wybar, K.C., Practical Orthoptics in the Treatment of Squint. H.K. Lewis & Co., London (1967).

Malbran, J., Strabismes et Paralysies. Héraly, Charleroi (1953).

von Noorden, G.K. und Maumenee, A.E., Atlas of Strabismus. The C.V. Mosby Company, St. Louis (1967).

Parks, M.M., Ocular Motility and Strabismus. Harper and Row, Hagerstown, Maryland (1975).

Sachsenweger, R., Augenmuskellähmungen. VEB Georg Thienne, Leipzig (1966).

Scobee, R.G., The Oculorotory Muscles. The C.V. Mosby Company, St. Louis (1952).

INDEX

Numbers in *italics* indicate
illustrations; numbers followed by t
indicate tables.